THE
COVID-19
Vaccine Guide

THE
COVID-19
Vaccine Guide

THE QUEST FOR IMPLEMENTATION OF SAFE AND EFFECTIVE VACCINATIONS

KATHRYN M. EDWARDS, MD,
WALTER A. ORENSTEIN, MD, DSc (Hon),
DAVID S. STEPHENS, MD

Skyhorse Publishing

Skyhorse Publishing books may be purchased in bulk at special discounts for sales promotion, corporate gifts, fund-raising, or educational purposes. Special editions can also be created to specifications. For details, contact the Special Sales Department, Skyhorse Publishing, 307 West 36th Street, 11th Floor, New York, NY 10018 or info@skyhorsepublishing.com.

Skyhorse® and Skyhorse Publishing® are registered trademarks of Skyhorse Publishing, Inc.®, a Delaware corporation.

Visit our website at www.skyhorsepublishing.com.

10 9 8 7 6 5 4 3 2 1

Library of Congress Cataloging-in-Publication Data is available on file.

Cover design by Laura Klynstra

Image Credits:

Cover image – ©2021 Emory University, created by Satyen Tripathi, MA CMI

Figure 1 – Orenstein WA, Ahmed R. Simply put: Vaccination saves lives. Proc. Natl. Acad. Sci. U.S.A. 2017;114(16):4031-4033 – Copyright (2017) National Academy of Sciences

Figure 2 – Provided by Destefano F, Immunization Safety Office, Centers for Disease Control and Prevention. Website: www.cdc.gov/vaccinesafety/iso.html.

Figures 3a & b – From Georgia Department of Public Health. Website: https://dph.georgia.gov/covid-19-daily-status-report.

Figure 4 – ©2021 Emory University, created by Michael Konomos

Figures 5a & b – ©2021 Emory University, created by Michael Konomos

Figure 6 – ©2021 Emory University, created by Michael Konomos

Figure 7 – Reprinted by permission from Macmillan Publishers Ltd: Nature. Callaway E. The race for coronavirus vaccines: a graphical guide. Nature 2020; 580:576. Copyright © 2020. https://www.nature.com/.
    Reproduced with permission from: Coronavirus disease 2019 (COVID-19): Vaccines to prevent SARS-CoV-2 infection. In: UpToDate, Post TW (Ed), UpToDate, Waltham, MA. (Accessed on 2/2/2021.) Copyright © 2021 UpToDate, Inc. For more information visit www.uptodate.com.

Figure 8 – Source: Institute for Health Metrics and Evaluation. Used with permission. All rights reserved.

Tables 1a & 1b – Provided by Roush S, Centers for Disease Control and Prevention.

Table 2 – From Centers for Disease Control and Prevention. Website: www.cdc.gov/vaccines/schedules/downloads/child/0-18yrs-child-combined-schedule.pdf.

Table 3 – From Centers for Disease Control and Prevention. Website: www.cdc.gov/vaccines/covid-19/info-by-product/clinical-considerations.html.

Print ISBN: 978-1-5107-6722-5
Ebook ISBN: 978-1-5107-6762-1

Printed in the United States of America

Contents

Contents

Dedication

This book is dedicated to the thousands of volunteers from many diverse backgrounds who enrolled in COVID-19 vaccine clinical trials in 2020. These individuals, through a commitment to research and to public health, facilitated emergency use authorization of safe and effective COVID-19 vaccines by the United States FDA and other regulatory agencies in less than one year. The book is also dedicated to the individuals who conducted the critically important foundational work on viruses including coronaviruses and the vaccine platforms that have been adapted to fight this pandemic. Also, to the vaccine developers and manufacturers who responded within days to the call to develop and manufacture COVID-19 vaccines, and to the private and governmental funding agencies that invested billions of dollars in this effort. In addition, thanks to the frontline workers and clinical coordinators from academic medical centers and from clinical research organizations who day by day and night by night performed and documented these clinical trials amid a raging pandemic. These contributions often go unrecognized. Finally, to the people who are diligently working to assure vaccines are distributed, delivered, and administered to persons for whom they are recommended. Only vaccinations, not vaccines, can stop this pandemic.

We also dedicate this work to the millions of individuals infected, the lives lost, and the suffering and pain inflicted by this pandemic. These individuals have also contributed to our understanding of COVID-19 and the imperative to prevention. The hope as a global society is that we forever recognize and prepare for future pandemics.

Chapter 1

COVID-19
Introduction and Illness

W e live in a microbial world. In December 2019, the Wuhan Municipal Health Committee, Hubei province, China, identified an outbreak of rapidly progressive and sometimes fatal viral pneumonia found to be due to a novel coronavirus named **Severe Acute Respiratory Syndrome CoronaVirus 2 (SARS-CoV-2)**. Since then the virus and the associated disease it causes, Coronavirus Disease 2019 (COVID-19), have rapidly spread globally, resulting in an unprecedented pandemic, not seen since the influenza pandemic of 1918–1919. COVID-19, transmitted from one person to another by respiratory droplets containing a highly infectious virus, is an acute infectious disease with variable respiratory and systemic manifestations. Most individuals have asymptomatic disease or mild or moderate disease. However, individuals over 65 years old and those with underlying health problems such as obesity, lung disease, cancer, chronic hypertension and heart disease, diabetes, kidney disease, and other chronic medical conditions are at greater risk for severe disease.

It also disproportionately affects populations of color. Progression to severe infection in the lungs leads to pneumonia and acute respiratory distress syndrome (ARDS), with subsequent failure of other organs and death. As of the end of February 2021, there were over 110 million confirmed cases of COVID-19 and approaching 2.5 million deaths worldwide with cases reported in every country and region around the world including Antarctica. However, this is the "tip of the iceberg." A conservative estimate is that five times as many infections have occurred than the cases reported with the number of reported deaths also a significant underestimate.

As this pandemic emerged and spread in early 2020, there was no vaccine against SARS-CoV-2. The unprecedented global effort to develop, manufacture, and deploy vaccines to prevent this disease is a part of the story in this book. By the end of January 2021, 237 COVID-19 vaccines were in development, and 63 of these were in human clinical trials.[1]

Currently, two COVID-19 vaccines made by Pfizer-BioNTech and Moderna have emergency use authorization (EUA) in the United States and Europe and one or both of these vaccines are being deployed in several other countries (the United Kingdom, Argentina, Chile, Bahrain, Canada, Saudi Arabia, Switzerland Singapore, and Israel). Other vaccines produced by Oxford-AstraZeneca and Johnson & Johnson (Janssen) have completed large-scale (phase 3) clinical trials, released efficacy results, and are authorized for use in several countries (the United Kingdom, Argentina, India, and Mexico); and one other manufacturer,

1   "Draft Landscape and Tracker of COVID-19 Candidate Vaccines." World Health Organization, January 26, 2021. https://www.who.int/publications/m/item/draft-landscape-of-covid-19-candidate-vaccines.

Novavax, has completed (and released initial efficacy results) and is conducting additional phase 3 trials. The phase 3 vaccine studies have shown very high protection against death, hospitalization, and severe illness. In addition, COVID-19 vaccines have been developed and clinically tested in China (Sinopharm, Sinovac, CanSino), Russia (Gamaleya Research Institute, Vector Institute), and India (Bharat Biotech) and these are being deployed in several countries. This is a remarkable and unprecedented accomplishment of science and medicine to have vaccines available and in use less than one year from identification of the outbreak.

COVID-19, THE ILLNESS

The first reports of SARS-CoV-2–infected individuals from China suggested that most COVID-19 cases were only mildly to moderately ill, with about 15% of the cases severe and 5% critical. As more experience was gained with COVID-19, the presentation of the infection can be divided into five stages. The **asymptomatic or presymptomatic stage** is characterized by detection of the virus in the nose and upper respiratory tract without any symptoms. Initially, the importance of asymptomatic infection was not appreciated. However, it was later found that many asymptomatic individuals were discovered to be infectious and could infect others. Unlike some other serious coronaviruses, individuals with SARS-CoV-2 are infectious before symptoms begin. Some individuals remain asymptomatic throughout the entire course of infection, while others progress to the further stages.

Symptomatic COVID-19 can be divided into different presentations. Mild COVID-19 (although many who have had the disease feel the term "mild" is a misnomer) is characterized by fever, cough, loss of taste or smell, but with no difficulty breathing. **Moderate COVID-19** is described as having symptoms of pneumonia such as high fever, worsening cough and shortness of breath on exertion, but still having normal levels of oxygen in the blood. **Severe COVID-19** is defined as having an increased rate of breathing at rest, decreased levels of oxygen in the blood, and evidence from X-rays or other chest scans that extensive pneumonia is present in the lungs. The most advanced stage of disease is termed **"Critical"** and is designated when there is failure of the lungs to provide adequate oxygen to the blood with the concurrent failure of other organ systems. At the onset of the outbreak it was projected that the fatality rate was between 1–3%, but with the detection of asymptomatic individuals and improved care, the overall fatality rate has decreased. However, the COVID-19 fatality rate is also dependent on age, with a much higher mortality rate in the elderly (those over 65 years). Also, mortality is greater in men than women, and higher mortality is seen in individuals with other medical conditions, as outlined above. Race and ethnicity are often markers for underlying conditions that affect health including socioeconomic status, access to healthcare, and exposure to the virus related to occupation (e.g., frontline, essential, and critical infrastructure workers). American Indians, Alaska Natives, Black or African Americans, and Hispanic or Latino persons have a 2.6–2.8× greater risk of death from COVID-19 than white non-hispanic populations.[2]

---

2 "COVID-19 Hospitalization and Death by Race/Ethnicity." Centers for Disease Control and Prevention, November 30, 2020. https://www.cdc .gov/coronavirus/2019-ncov/covid-data/investigations-discovery/ hospitalization-death-by-race-ethnicity.html.

Symptoms of COVID-19

Fever and chills are a prominent feature of COVID-19 illness. Initially fever is present in approximately 60% of individuals and is 100.4°F or higher at onset. Over the subsequent course of the disease, fever occurs in 83–99%, but the temperature is variable with nearly 20% having only an initial low-grade fever <100.4°F. A new or increased cough is seen in nearly 60% at onset, and over 80% develop cough over the course of illness. Generally, at least one additional symptom develops from the following list:

- Fatigue/profound weakness occurs in about 70% (at onset and over course of the illness; this often lasts for two or three weeks)
- New loss of taste and/or smell occurs in two-thirds or more (onset early in the illness and is a characteristic symptom of COVID-19)
- Severe headache occurs in about 40% (often at onset)

Other less specific symptoms include:

- Loss of appetite (anorexia) occurs in 40–84%, and gastro-intestinal symptoms, nausea, and vomiting in 10–30%
- Myalgias (muscle pain) occurs in about 35%
- Sore throat and initial runny nose are less common

Shortness of breath or difficulty breathing occurs in 40% and can progress in the later stages of disease. Persistent pain or pressure in the chest can emerge four to 10 days after onset of illness in a subset of those infected. X-rays, as noted, show "diffuse pulmonary infiltrates" or pneumonia throughout the lung (pneumonia is often best seen on a chest computerized tomography CAT scan. There is evidence of lack of oxygen (hypoxia) with low oxygen (O_2) saturation in the blood, that is, an O_2 saturation of <94%. As noted below, clotting of the blood is an important complication in some individuals, called "thromboembolic" complications. Failure of the lungs to deliver oxygen to the blood may necessitate mechanical ventilation. Respiratory failure and severe inflammation in the lungs and bloodstream (cytokine storm) can lead to death.

The virus spreads from the initial site of entry in the nose and upper respiratory tract to the lungs, causing the pneumonia. It can also be found in the gastrointestinal tract. The virus also may spread to other organs or more commonly induce in the lungs and blood the inflammatory response that causes neurologic, heart (cardiac), kidney (renal), and skin involvement. Again, one of the most prominent aspects of severe COVID-19 is the tendency to cause blood clots throughout the body, including the brain, lungs, kidneys, and heart. Severely ill hospitalized patients have fever, increased blood proteins that promote blood clotting, and evidence of inflammation in all the organs of the body. In an autopsy study of people who have died from COVID-19, the lungs showed blood clots and inflammation.

Some individuals, maybe up to 10% of those infected, who recover from COVID-19 have persistent symptoms, the "COVID-19 long-hauler syndrome." We are still learning about the spectrum of conditions associated with this syndrome. Symptoms include persistent cough, persistent fatigue, chronic shortness of breath, cardiac dysfunction ("cardiomyopathy"), memory loss or inability to concentrate, difficulty sleeping, headaches, and joint pain.

Children have lower rates of COVID-19 incidence and hospitalization. Clinical symptoms in children are less severe than those seen in adults with more asymptomatic infections and milder cases. This is distinctly different from other respiratory infections, such as influenza or respiratory syncytial virus, where children have more severe symptoms than adults. However, some children, particularly adolescents and older children with comorbidities such as obesity, can have a critical course with mortality. Children have also developed a later disease called multisystem inflammatory syndrome in children (MIS-C) 2–6 weeks after COVID-19 infection. These children have varied clinical manifestations but these include high fever, rash, abdominal pain, and heart failure. If this condition is promptly managed with medications to support the heart and reduce the inflammation, the children generally do well. The disparities by race and ethnicity noted among COVID-19 adults are also seen in children.

COVID-19 in pregnant women is usually associated with a low risk for transmission to the infant while in utero. A few pregnant women have a more complicated course with pneumonia, organ dysfunction, and premature delivery. SARS-CoV-2 virus is not detected in breast milk, and infants can be breastfed. Infected mothers need to practice masking and careful handwashing to prevent transmission of the virus to the infant after birth.

Chapter 2

Introduction to Vaccines and Vaccinology

Vaccines are the most cost-effective intervention for preventing human disease. What is a vaccine? How does it work? How do vaccines protect?

A vaccine is a substance, such as an inactivated protein from an infectious organism, that when given to a person induces an active immune response to prevent or mitigate a disease. Your immune system acts as an army. The immune system ideally detects the foreign invading germ (i.e., virus, bacterium, fungus), generally called a "pathogen," and destroys it or contains it so that it cannot cause disease. What a vaccine does is give the immune system practice so that when it encounters the real pathogen, it is ready. Without practice from the vaccine, the pathogen can overwhelm an unprepared immune system, causing serious illness.

The immune system can protect against infection and disease in two different ways. First, it can secrete immune proteins, called antibodies, into blood or tissues that bind to the invading pathogen and prevent it from multiplying or invading cells of the human body and enhancing the uptake of the pathogens into special cells ("phagocytes") which destroy the pathogen. This aspect of the immune system is often called the humoral immune system. Critical players in this response are B cells and specialized B cells called plasma cells. The plasma cells produce the antibodies that circulate in the blood and other body fluids and tissues, which when encountering the pathogen neutralize it or bind to it, facilitating destruction of the pathogen by other cells of the immune system.

Second, the immune system consists of specialized cells, called T cells, which destroy infected human cells and prevent the pathogen from spreading and causing serious disease. This aspect of the immune system is called the cellular immune system.

A number of vaccines include substances called adjuvants or immune system helpers. These adjuvants enhance the immune response to the vaccine. In the United States, the most common adjuvants are aluminum-based compounds. But an increasing number of vaccines have other new adjuvants that stimulate immunity, particularly in the elderly or those with less-robust immune responses (see https://www.cdc.gov/vaccinesafety/concerns/adjuvants.html).

The first vaccine was developed in 1796 by William Jenner. He had noticed that milkmaids in the United Kingdom did not get smallpox. He also noted that many of them had mild skin lesions, called cowpox, from which they had recovered without serious illness. He hypothesized that cowpox infection led to protection from smallpox. On May 14, 1796, he inoculated James Phipps, a child, with pus from a milkmaid, Sarah Nelms. After James recovered from the cowpox, Jenner exposed him to smallpox and the child was protected. The cowpox virus was later named "vaccinia" after the Latin word for cow, *vacca*, which later became the root of the word "vaccine."

There are many types of vaccines. The first vaccines developed were modeled on those of Jenner and included related viruses or bacteria that infected animals and were able to induce cross-protective immunity against human pathogens, when injected into humans. Examples of these vaccines include the previously mentioned smallpox vaccine used by Jenner and another animal bacteria from cows, called BCG, that is administered to children in developing countries to protect against tuberculosis. Next came killed whole viruses or bacteria with an excellent example being the inactivated or killed polio vaccine (IPV) developed by Jonas Salk, which became available in 1955. Another vaccine in this category includes a virus to prevent hepatitis (inflammation of the liver) called hepatitis A.

Some bacteria cause disease by excreting potent substances, called toxins, into the body. There are ways to chemically alter these toxins so they no longer cause disease but do stimulate a protective immune response. These are called "toxoids" and the major examples of these are toxoids to prevent tetanus and diphtheria, which are given as part of the combined diphtheria, tetanus, and pertussis (DTP) vaccine. Another example of the use of proteins released from an organism to produce vaccines is the acellular pertussis or whooping cough vaccine, which contains several of these purified proteins from the pathogen (called *Bordetella pertussis*) and used as a vaccine.

A major breakthrough in vaccinology came with the development of live attenuated or weakened pathogens that through repeated passage in the laboratory lost their virulence but maintained their ability to induce a protective immune response. Examples of these vaccines include those against measles, mumps, rubella, varicella (chickenpox), and yellow fever. The organisms in these vaccines can reproduce in the body following administration, cause the immune system to recognize them as foreign, and thereby induce the immune system to make and sustain a protective immune response.

Some bacteria have capsules made of complex sugars, called polysaccharides, to protect the bacteria. Another class of vaccines induce the immune system to make antibodies against these polysaccharides and protect the body from diseases these bacteria cause. Sometimes these polysaccharides do not induce a protective immune response by themselves, particularly in young children. But when the polysaccharides are chemically linked to proteins, they become better able to stimulate a potent immune response. These are called protein-polysaccharide conjugate vaccines. Examples of such vaccines are the pneumococcal conjugate vaccine, which protects against common causes of severe pneumonia and the meningococcal conjugate vaccines that protect against epidemic meningitis.

Another major breakthrough in the field of vaccinology has been the production of particles that look like the surface of a given pathogen. These vaccines are made by taking a gene from the pathogen, which often codes for a part of the surface of that pathogen, and putting it into another organism, which expresses and excretes the protein. When excreted, the protein forms particles with the surface similar to the surface of the pathogen. These particles are then purified and can become vaccines, inducing an active immune response against the original pathogen. An example of this technology is the hepatitis B vaccine. Hepatitis B is a virus that can cause liver inflammation, fibrosis (cirrhosis) of the liver, and liver cancer. Another example is the human papilloma virus (HPV) vaccine, which is highly effective in preventing cervical cancer and several other types of cancer caused by HPV.

Some vaccines are made through taking a virus that is generally not harmful and inserting a critical gene that codes for part of another pathogen into that virus. The virus carrying this gene is called a vector. This technique uses a viral vector or carrier as a Trojan horse to introduce a critical gene from another pathogen to stimulate immunity. When administered to humans, the vector virus enters the body and produces the protein that is recognized as foreign by the immune system, which in turn makes a protective immune response. Examples of this include an Ebola vaccine that uses a relatively harmless virus called the vesicular stomatitis virus as the vector and inserts a gene for the surface of the Ebola virus into the virus. This leads to vesicular stomatitis virus expressing the Ebola protein for which that gene codes, on its surface. When the immune system interacts with this foreign protein it makes a protective immune response against the protein. Thus, should the vaccinee later be exposed to Ebola virus, the immune system is ready and destroys the Ebola virus before it can cause disease.

Another technique has been to take a weakened virus or a virus that infects an animal or animals but does not cause disease in humans and incubate or culture the virus in the laboratory with a virus that causes human disease. When the viruses both infect a cell in the laboratory at the same time, they can exchange genes. Thus, the gene coding for a surface component of the human disease-causing pathogen may replace the same gene in the weakened virus. When this weakened "reassortant" virus is given to humans it can induce protective immunity against the surface component of the human disease-causing pathogen without causing disease. Examples of this technology include a live influenza vaccine administered into the nose and a vaccine that protects against rotavirus, a common cause of severe diarrhea in children.

The new techniques applicable to COVID-19 vaccines will be discussed in **Chapter 3**.

As noted earlier in this chapter, vaccines induce individual protection by inducing protective immune responses. Most vaccines also induce **community protection**, often called **"herd or population immunity."** Since most vaccine-preventable diseases result from person-to-person spread, when an individual is infected, the pathogen reproduces in that person's body and then spreads from the infected person to others. When the infectious person encounters a susceptible individual, the infectious person can transmit the infection. The cycle can then be repeated by infecting another contact, which is known as a **chain of transmission**. However, if the infectious person encounters an immune individual, there is no (or perhaps very limited) transmission. If a high percentage of the population is immune to the infection, then transmission does not occur, and the chain of human-to-human transmission is broken (Figure 1, page 15).

Figure 1

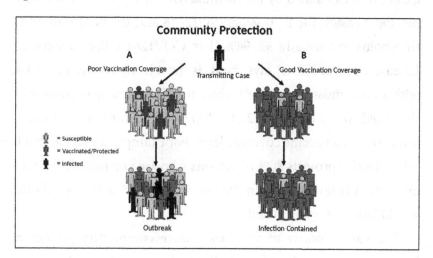

No individual has infinite contacts. Mathematical modelers can review the epidemiology of a given disease and calculate a number called the **basic reproduction number or R_0** (called R naught). The R_0 is the average number of persons an infected individual would subsequently infect if they lived in a community in which 100% of the people living in that community were susceptible. The immunity level needed in a community to stop transmission is called the "herd immunity threshold." For example, if R_0 was 4, then the average transmitting case would infect four people if they lived in a community that was 100% susceptible to the infection. If the immunity level in that community was 75%, then of the four contacts of the infectious case, three would be immune. Thus, in that situation, the average transmitter would infect one person and the level of disease would remain constant. If the immunity level went above 75%, then the average transmitter would infect <1 person and transmission would die out. The herd immunity threshold for a disease is calculated by the formula $((R_0-1)/R_0) \times 100$. For example, for measles, the R_0 is generally 12–18 and the herd immunity thresholds are usually 92–94%. For COVID-19, the Centers for Disease Control (CDC) says the R_0 is most likely between 2 and 4, with 2.5 the most likely case[1]). Thus, if R_0 is 2.5, the herd immunity threshold would be $(2.5-1)/2.5) \times 100$ or 60%. This is an immunity level and not a vaccine coverage level. For example, a vaccine that is 80% effective protects 80% of persons who are vaccinated. To reach an immunity level of 60% in the population, 75% of the population would have to be vaccinated.

The vast majority of vaccines induce community protection because they not only protect individuals exposed to an infectious pathogen from getting ill but they also prevent such persons from transmitting the pathogen to others who are susceptible. Thus, a goal for many vaccination programs is to induce immunity levels greater than the herd immunity threshold to terminate disease risk in that community. Therefore, 100% immunity is not needed to stop transmission. Vaccines that prevent transmission as well as disease protect the community at large. The need for indirect protection is greatest in those individuals who cannot be effectively vaccinated and include: 1) children too young to be vaccinated against a specific disease; 2) persons who have legitimate medical contraindications to vaccination; and 3) persons, usually a small percentage, who fail to make a protective immune response after vaccination.

---

1   "COVID-19 Pandemic Planning Scenarios." Centers for Disease Control and Prevention, September 10, 2020. https://www.cdc.gov/coronavirus /2019-ncov/hcp/planning-scenarios.html#five-scenarios.

THE REMARKABLE IMPACT OF VACCINES ON HUMAN HEALTH

Few measures in modern medicine can compare with the impact of vaccines in reducing health burdens and preventing disease (Tables 1a and b). Advantages of vaccines include the fact that most are highly safe and effective. Further, for many vaccines, one needs to have only a limited number of doses for protection. In contrast, prevention of many other diseases, particularly chronic diseases, requires lifetime changes in behavior or chronic medication receipt.

The only human disease ever eradicated, smallpox, was eradicated using a vaccine. In the early 20th century, about 29,000 cases of smallpox were reported each year in the United States alone. Smallpox, the major variety of which was known as variola major, was associated with about a 30% case-fatality rate. Smallpox was declared officially eradicated in 1980 with the last cases in the world in the United Kingdom in 1978 that resulted from exposure to smallpox virus in a laboratory accident. There have been no cases of smallpox anywhere in the world since the 1978 accident, an incredible scientific and public health achievement.

Another major vaccine triumph came from development of a live attenuated (weakened) measles vaccine, which became available in the United States in 1963. Prior to availability of measles vaccine, an estimated four million measles cases occurred each year in the United States leading to 48,000 hospitalizations and several hundred deaths/year. While measles has not been eradicated from the world, the measles virus is no longer circulating in the United States. The United States was certified as having eliminated indigenous measles virus in 2000. However, vaccination must continue, because measles has not been eliminated in much of the world, leading to the ongoing threat of imported measles in the United States, leading to outbreaks. In fact, the number of cases reported in 2019 was the largest number since 1992. Fortunately, transmission of measles viruses in the United States in 2019 was stopped, meaning the circulation in the country did not exceed a year. If it had, the United States would have lost its measles elimination status.

Another major vaccine success was the development of a live attenuated rubella vaccine. During the 1964–1965 rubella pandemic, an estimated 20,000 children were born with congenital rubella syndrome, often causing deafness, blindness, mental retardation, and other severe abnormalities. Infection of pregnant women with rubella virus is a known cause of autism. With use of the rubella vaccine, the United States eliminated transmission in the country and in recent years there have not been any cases of congenital rubella among children whose mothers were US residents.

Polio is a terrible disease. During the early 1950s, about 20,000 persons a year were paralyzed by the poliovirus. The poliovirus attacked cells of the central nervous system and spinal cord which control muscle function. When the virus destroyed the nerves to limb muscles, persons were paralyzed, mostly for life. If the virus destroyed the nerves to respiratory muscles, breathing could stop, leading to death. The development and widespread uptake first of the killed inactivated poliovirus (IPV) developed by Jonas Salk, followed by development by Albert Sabin of a live attenuated or weakened poliovirus administered orally, led to elimination of polio in the United States. The last polio outbreak in the United States due to wild poliovirus occurred in 1979. The world is now close to eradicating polio as it did with smallpox, using polio vaccines. In the United States today, we use an enhanced-potency IPV.

Another vaccine with a major impact is that against *Haemophilus influenzae* type b, better known as Hib. This bacterium causes severe invasive disease including meningitis leading to brain damage, pneumonia, bloodstream infections, and more. Prior to vaccination, there were an estimated 20,000 cases of invasive Hib disease annually, including about 12,000 cases of meningitis in the United States. As physicians during the pre-vaccine era, we remember the repeated spinal taps on children suspected to have Hib meningitis, confirming the infection, and starting intravenous lines and antibiotics to attempt to cure or ameliorate the disease. Today, most young pediatricians have never seen a case of Hib meningitis because of widespread vaccination with Hib vaccine. The Hib vaccine is made from a complex sugar (polysaccharide) covering the organism, which is chemically linked to a protein to enhance its immunogenicity. The Hib vaccine also has played a major role in inducing community protection through marked reductions in the circulation of the bacterium.

Other vaccine successes have included the development of vaccines that can prevent cancer. Hepatitis B virus (HepB) is a major cause of liver cancer. Human papilloma virus (HPV) is a major cause of cervical cancer, oropharyngeal cancer, and many more cancers. The vaccines we have against these viruses prevent cancer by preventing the chronic infection caused by these viruses. The vaccines stimulate our immune systems to destroy these viruses before they infect us.

The list of vaccine-preventable diseases is fortunately long and getting longer. As of 2020, all children without medical contraindications to the vaccines are recommended to be vaccinated against 16 diseases. These diseases include diphtheria, tetanus, pertussis (whooping cough), polio, rotavirus, pneumococcal disease, Hib, hepatitis A, hepatitis B, measles, mumps, rubella, varicella (chickenpox), influenza, meningococcal disease, and HPV. The childhood immunization schedule is shown in Table 2 (page 23)[2].

All adults are recommended to be vaccinated against at least three diseases: pneumococcal disease, influenza, and shingles (Herpes Zoster).

Recommendations for vaccinations for children and adults are updated annually and can be found at: https://www.cdc.gov/vaccines/schedules/hcp/index.html.

In addition to vaccines routinely recommended for all children and/or adults without medical contraindications, there are many other vaccines available for people in special situations such as foreign travel. Information on vaccines is available at: https://www.cdc.gov/vaccines/hcp/acip-recs/index.html.

---

2   "Recommended Child and Adolescent Immunization Schedule for Ages 18 Years or Younger." Centers for Disease Control and Prevention, February 16, 2021. www.cdc.gov/vaccines/schedules/hcp/imz/child-adolescent.html.

Table 1a.

Comparison of 20th-Century Annual Morbidity and Current Estimates Vaccine-Preventable Diseases

Disease	20th Century Annual Morbidity †	2019 Reported Percent ††	Percent Decrease
Smallpox	29,005	0	100%
Diphtheria	21,053	1	> 99%
Measles	530,217	13	> 99%
Mumps	162,344	621	99%
Pertussis	200,752	5,398	97%
Polio (paralytic)	16,316	0	100%
Rubella	47,745	6	> 99%
Congenital Rubella Syndrome	152	0	100%
Tetanus	580	15	97%
Haemophilus influenzae	20,000	11*	> 99%

† *JAMA*. 2007;298(18):2155–2163.

††CDC. *National Notifiable Diseases Surveillance System, Weekly Tables of Infectious Disease Data*. Atlanta, GA. CDC Division of Health Informatics and Surveillance. Available at: https://wonder.cdc.gov/nndss/nndss_weekly_tables_menu.asp?mmwr _year=2020&mmwr_week=53.

* *Haemophilus influenzae* type b (Hib) < 5 years of age. An additional 7 cases of Hib are estimated to have occurred among the 136 notifications of Hib (< 5 years of age) with unknown serotype.

Data provided by S. Roush, CDC, via email January 1, 2021.

Table 1b.

Comparison of Pre-Vaccine–Era Estimated Annual Morbidity with Current Estimate: Vaccine-Preventable Diseases

Disease	Pre-Vaccine Era Annual Estimate †	2016 Estimate (unless other-wise specified)	Percent Decrease
Hepatitis A	117,333 †	4,000 *	97%
Hepatitis B (acute)	66,232†	20,900 *	68%
Pneumococcus (invasive) all ages / < 5 years of age	63,067 † / 16,069 †	30,400 # / 1,700 #	52% / 89%
Rotavirus (hospitalizations, < 3 years of age)	62,500 ††	30,625 ##	51%
Varicella	4,085,120 †	102,128 ###	98%

† JAMA. 2007;298(18):2155–2163.

† † CDC. MMWR. February 6, 2009 / 58(RR02);1–25.

* CDC. Viral Hepatitis Surveillance—United States, 2016.

CDC. Unpublished, Active Bacterial Core Surveillance, 2016.

New Vaccine Surveillance Network 2017 data (unpublished); U.S. rotavirus disease now has biennial pattern.

CDC. Varicella Program 2017 data (unpublished).

Data provided by S. Roush, CDC, via email January 11, 2019.

Table 2.

Recommended Child and Adolescent Immunization Schedule for Ages 18 Years or Younger, United States, 2021[3]

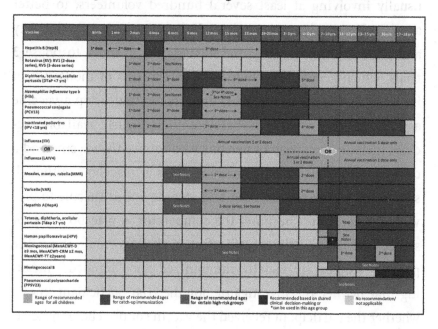

For the most up-to-date immunization schedules go to www.cdc.gov/vaccines/schedules/.

CRITICAL STAGES IN VACCINE DEVELOPMENT

A critical part of developing a vaccine is to demonstrate the efficacy and safety of the vaccine through a set of clinical trials in humans, spanning phase 1 through phase 3 trials. Phase 1 "first in humans" trials generally include 20–100 volunteers with a primary goal of determining the appropriate dosing to induce an immune

---

3   "Recommended Child and Adolescent Immunization Schedule for Ages 18 Years or Younger." Centers for Disease Control and Prevention, February 16, 2021. www.cdc.gov/vaccines/schedules/hcp/imz/child-adolescent.html.

response thought to be protective (immunogenic) as well as to begin to evaluate vaccine safety. If the results support that the vaccine is immunogenic and safe, then phase 2 trials are conducted, usually involving at least several hundred volunteers, to better assess safety and immunogenicity. If those trials show both safety and good immunogenicity, the next step is to move to phase 3 trials, which generally include hundreds to tens of thousands of individuals. Most phase 3 trials undertaken to develop a vaccine against a disease for which there are no previously available vaccines include one group of persons who receive the vaccine and a comparator group, which usually receives a "placebo"—although sometimes an already licensed and recommended vaccine to prevent another illness becomes the comparator. A placebo is a substance that has no therapeutic effect, such as normal saline. The phase 3 studies are usually randomized and "blinded," meaning that neither the investigator nor the trial participant knows whether the participant received the vaccine or placebo. Efficacy is measured as a percentage and is measured by comparing the rate of disease in vaccinees versus placebo recipients and is calculated by the following formula: $((ARU-ARV)/ARU)) \times 100$. ARU is the attack rate in the unvaccinated and ARV is the attack rate in the vaccinated group. For example, if the attack rate in placebo recipients of a given disease is 80% and the attack rate in vaccinees is 40%, then the vaccine efficacy is 50%. In other words, vaccination will reduce the risk of getting disease by 50% compared to people who are unvaccinated.

A goal is to learn whether there is a **correlate of protection**, for example an antibody level that if achieved can be assumed to provide protection. Such correlates may be obtained in initial clinical trials or after vaccine approval and are determined from individuals in which the vaccine does not prevent disease. For example, there should be no disease in persons who achieve the presumed correlate of protection (e.g., antibody level). In contrast, persons who fail to achieve such an antibody level can get the infection. Getting a correlate of protection from initial clinical trials can facilitate future trials because investigators do not have to wait to see the incidence of disease in the trial population among vaccinees versus non-vaccinees. They can simply look at the proportion of vaccinees who make that antibody level or the "immune correlate of protection" and assume that the efficacy will correlate with the proportion making that antibody level.

Safety evaluation is a critical part of vaccine development. Adverse events are compared between the persons in the vaccine arm versus the placebo arm. If the rate of specific adverse events or clinical syndromes in the group receiving the placebo is the same as in the vaccine group, then the implication is the events are coincidental and not causally related to the vaccine. On the other hand, if the specific adverse event is significantly higher in the vaccine group than the placebo group, this would suggest the event is causally related to the vaccine. Further, by comparing the rates of the adverse event in vaccinees versus placebo recipients, one can calculate the rate attributable to the vaccine. For example, if the rate of adverse event A is 5 per 1,000 in the vaccine recipients and 1 per 1,000 in placebo recipients, then the risk of vaccine causing the syndrome is 5/1,000 minus 1/1,000 or 4 per 1,000 vaccine recipients (1 in 250 vaccinees).

The critical role of regulatory agencies such as the United States Food and Drug Administration (FDA) in the approval of vaccines to be used in the population

The Center for Biologics Evaluation and Research (CBER) is the critical group within FDA that licenses vaccines for use in the United States. Full licensure of vaccines requires a comprehensive process and detailed review to assure vaccines are both safe and effective. Vaccine developers perform preclinical work in cells, small animals, and other models to identify dose and potential safety concerns, to assess the immune response associated with protection in these models, and to assess what may constitute a protective immune response. This is done in animals including nonhuman primates and includes assessments of safety and of antibody levels attained as well as cell-mediated (T cell) immune responses. Further, the potential manufacturer must develop a reliable manufacturing process to produce the vaccine that can be used in clinical trials. During preclinical testing, and when the manufacturing process and preliminary preclinical data are being completed, manufacturers develop a protocol and approach the FDA for permission to enter human clinical trials. The sponsor of the trial seeks approval through a detailed and iterative process of an Investigational New Drug application, or IND, from the FDA to begin human clinical trials.

In the application for an IND, the sponsor describes: 1) the composition, source, and method of manufacturing and the methods used to test its safety, purity, and potency; 2) a summary of all laboratory and preclinical testing in animals; and 3) the plan to evaluate the product including details of the clinical study or studies and the names and qualifications of the investigators who will conduct the human clinical studies. A consent form that will have to be signed by participants in the study must be developed. An institutional review board (IRB) at each of the sites where the research will be performed must review and approve the consent form. If all the required guidelines are met and questions addressed, then the FDA will issue an IND and the study can begin.

The clinical trials are described in the section titled "Critical Stages in Vaccine Development" (page 23). Following completion of the phase 3 trial, and if the results show the vaccine is both safe and effective, the sponsor of the trial submits a Biologics License Application (BLA) to the FDA for review and approval. In addition to including results of the clinical trial in the BLA, it is critical to detail the manufacturing process. This includes information on organization and personnel, equipment used, buildings and facilities, control of components and containers, production and process controls, packaging and labeling controls, holding and distribution, laboratory controls, and records to be maintained. In addition, the sponsor must provide a full description of the manufacturing methods, information supporting stability of the vaccine, and duration of time the product would be considered effective. The manufacturer must prepare several batches of the vaccine to prove to the FDA that the process is consistent and reproducible.

The BLA also should include proposed product labeling including indications for use, vaccination schedules, contraindications, dosage, possible adverse events, and protocols for testing lots to assure they are potent and not altered from the initial approved product. CBER then performs an internal scientific review of the

BLA, which can include communications with the sponsor for further information, clarifying information, and answering questions CBER reviewers pose. The review also includes a CBER inspection of the manufacturing facility to assure it complies with FDA requirements for production and distribution.

After CBER reviews the information above, it seeks guidance from its external advisory committee (Vaccines and Related Biological Products Advisory Committee [VRBPAC]) to assess whether the vaccine information provided shows that the product is both safe and effective and that the benefits of the vaccine outweigh any risks. VRBPAC consists of a core of 15 voting members including the chair. Members and the chair are selected by the commissioner or designee from among authorities knowledgeable in the fields of immunology, molecular biology, rDNA, virology, bacteriology, epidemiology or biostatistics, vaccine policy, vaccine safety science, federal immunization activities, vaccine development including translational and clinical evaluation programs, allergy, preventive medicine, infectious diseases, pediatrics, microbiology, and biochemistry. The VRBPAC meeting presentations and meeting materials are public and meetings can be heard, viewed, captioned, and recorded through an online teleconferencing platform. VRBPAC advises the FDA commissioner or designee as they relate to helping to ensure safe and effective vaccines and related biological products for human use. The committee reviews and evaluates data concerning the safety, effectiveness, and appropriate use of vaccines and related biological products that are intended for use in the prevention, treatment, or diagnosis of human diseases, and, as required, any other products for which the FDA has regulatory responsibility. The committee also considers the quality and relevance of FDA's research program, which provides scientific support for the regulation of these products and makes appropriate recommendations to the FDA commissioner. Once the advisory committee recommendations are reviewed and approved by CBER, the product is licensed and may be manufactured and distributed for use.

As we have seen with COVID-19 vaccines, the FDA also has the ability to grant an emergency use authorization (EUA) for a product during a public health emergency when there are no licensed alternatives to meet the need to mitigate the public health problem.[4]

Under these circumstances, the FDA evaluates available data on safety, effectiveness, and manufacturing and judges that the benefits of the product under evaluation outweigh the risks, given the public health emergency. The FDA often seeks VRBPAC advice on issuance of an EUA for specific biological products including vaccines. Products available through EUAs are not considered licensed. The FDA requires special documents be created for persons using the product and for recipients of the product. Manufacturers prepare such documents, which are reviewed by the FDA.

Similar regulatory agencies are present globally. The European Medicines Agency (EMA) has responsibilities for authorizing and

---

4 Center for Biologics Evaluation and Research. "Emergency Use Authorization for Vaccines Explained." U.S. Food and Drug Administration. FDA, November 20, 2020. https://www.fda.gov/vaccines-blood-biologics/vaccines/emergency-use-authorization-vaccines-explained.

monitoring vaccines in the EU (European Union). The WHO also reviews and issues approvals for global distribution of vaccines.

The role of the United States CDC's Advisory Committee on Immunization Practices (ACIP) in making vaccine recommendations

National recommendations for vaccine distribution and use are separate from the regulatory approval of a vaccine. The ACIP is the major advisory group making recommendations for actual use of licensed or EUA vaccines in the United States. It was formed in 1964 and currently consists of 15 voting members who meet at least three times per year. ACIP members cannot be government employees and must declare any conflicts of interest (COI) they may have regarding a recommendation for a specific product. Should a member have a COI, they disclose and must abstain on any votes related to that product. In determining their recommendations, the ACIP considers the epidemiology of the disease to be prevented, including the burden of disease, vaccine effectiveness, vaccine safety, the quality of the evidence reviewed, economic analyses of the cost-effectiveness and benefit of various vaccination strategies, and the feasibility of implementing potential vaccine recommendations.

In addition to voting members, there are liaison representatives from many major medical organizations as well as ex officio representatives from other critical federal agencies, such as the FDA. These nonvoting members can participate in discussions of ACIP recommendations. ACIP meetings are conducted in public and anyone can listen in (see www.cdc.gov/vaccines/acip/index.html). Limited time is allotted in every ACIP meeting for public input.

Persons who do not have an opportunity to speak at the meeting can offer written comments for the committee to review.

The major work of the ACIP is accomplished through specific working groups. These groups, which consist of at least two ACIP voting members, include ACIP ex officio members, liaison members, and expert consultants. Staffing of the working groups is provided by CDC subject matter experts. The working groups review all the evidence noted above and synthesize potential recommendations for the whole ACIP to consider. A critical part of ACIP deliberations is evaluating the quality of the evidence used to develop recommendations. This process includes: Grading of Recommendations, Assessment, Development, and Evaluation (GRADE) (see www.cdc.gov/vaccines/acip/recs/). Another part of presentations by working groups to the whole ACIP is Evidence to Recommendations (EtR). Factors considered in EtR include: 1) the problem to be addressed by vaccination (Is it a public health problem?); 2) What are the benefits and harms of the vaccination strategy; 3) Values (Does the proposed target population for vaccination feel the desirable effects of the vaccine outweigh the undesirable?); 4) Acceptability (Is the intervention acceptable to key stakeholders?); 5) Resource use (Is the intervention a reasonable and efficient use of resources?); and 6) Feasibility (Is the intervention reasonable to implement?).

ACIP recommendations are developed based on majority votes. Once approved by the ACIP, they are sent to the CDC director, who must approve the recommendations before they are accepted and implemented. ACIP recommendations become official when published in the Morbidity and Mortality Weekly Report (MMWR).[5]

---

5 "ACIP Vaccine Recommendations." Centers for Disease Control and Prevention, July 16, 2013. https://www.cdc.gov/vaccines/hcp/acip-recs/index.html.

The ACIP plays a major role in recommending which groups should have priorities for vaccines when available supply is inadequate to cover all persons for whom the vaccine is recommended. Factors considered in the ACIP allocation priorities include: 1) decrease death and serious disease as much as possible; 2) preserve functioning of society; and 3) reduce the burden that the disease is having on people already facing disparities.[6] In addition, the ACIP is guided by ethical principles including: 1) maximize benefits and minimize harms; 2) mitigate health inequities; 3) promote justice; and 4) promote transparency.

For COVID-19 vaccines, the ACIP developed four phases of allocation of vaccines. The top priority, phase 1a, consists of healthcare personnel and residents of long-term care facilities. The next priority, phase 1b, includes frontline essential workers and persons 75 years of age and older. Frontline essential workers include: first responders (e.g., firefighters and police officers), corrections officers, food and agricultural workers, U.S. Postal Service workers, manufacturing workers, grocery store workers, public transit workers, and those who work in the education sector (teachers and support staff members) as well as childcare workers.[7]. The third priority, phase 1c, includes persons aged 65–74 years, persons aged 16–64 years with medical conditions that increase the risk for severe COVID-19, and essential workers not previously included

---

6 "How CDC Is Making COVID-19 Vaccine Recommendations." Centers for Disease Control and Prevention, December 30, 2020. https://www.cdc.gov/coronavirus/2019-ncov/vaccines/recommendations-process.html.

7 "The Advisory Committee on Immunization Practices' Updated Interim Recommendation for Allocation of COVID-19 Vaccine - United States, December 2020." Centers for Disease Control and Prevention, December 31, 2020. https://www.cdc.gov/mmwr/volumes/69/wr/mm695152e2.htm.

in phase 1a or 1b. The fourth priority group, phase 2, were all persons 16–64 years of age not included in phases 1a to 1c.

Other countries have established similar committees for national vaccine recommendations. In the United Kingdom, the Joint Committee on Vaccination and Immunization (JCVI) advises UK health departments on immunization.

Other factors critical to assuring access to safe and effective vaccines

First, distribution of vaccines must be done to ensure that when vaccines arrive at their intended destinations, they remain potent, stable, and safe. Most vaccines require adherence to strict temperature requirements during transport and storage. Monitoring is needed to assure vaccines stay at required temperatures. This is often called "maintaining the cold-chain." Further, once at their final destinations, vaccines must be maintained at the temperatures specified in the FDA-approved package inserts. Many vaccines consist of a freeze-dried portion in a vial, which is a solid. The vaccine comes with a separate vial containing a diluent. With a needle and syringe, the diluent is withdrawn from its vial and then injected into the vial containing the solid portion. This is then shaken until the solid dissolves. The volume of diluent to be used is specified in the package insert, and the person mixing the vaccine should not deviate from the recommended volume. The vial may contain multiple doses of vaccine. The vaccinator should remove with a needle and syringe only the volume needed for a single dose of the vaccine. The vaccinator should also follow the package insert instructions for where to administer the vaccine such as into muscle, into subcutaneous tissue, or orally, etc.

Many vials of vaccines, once reconstituted with diluent, must be discarded after a single vaccination session, even if there are still doses in those vials. A few vaccines have preservatives in them that allow storage for a longer period if temperature controls are maintained. The preservatives are designed to prevent overgrowth of bacteria, should they be inadvertently introduced during reconstitution or withdrawal of initial doses. Most vaccines in use in the United States do not have preservatives. A major exception is multi-dose vials of some influenza vaccines.

Other barriers to access include administering vaccines at locations that are inconvenient for potential vaccinees, hours that vaccines are available that interfere with other activities, such as work, and financial barriers to access. In the United States, attempts to minimize financial barriers to access for vaccines recommended for children include the Vaccines for Children Program (VFC). Children eligible for VFC include those with no insurance, children on Medicaid, and American Indians/Alaskan Natives. Children covered by VFC can receive vaccines free of charge, generally at their regular provider. The Affordable Care Act requires insurance companies to cover the full cost of vaccination for ACIP-recommended vaccines for persons who seek that care at an in-network provider. Other ways to minimize barriers include making vaccines available at convenient sites, such as pharmacies, instead of having to make an appointment and go to a physician's office.

The need for monitoring of vaccines and vaccination after manufacturers receive a license or an EUA

Many critical questions may not have been answered in studies or clinical trials of vaccines prior to licensure or granting of an EUA. For example, most clinical trials will not evaluate duration of immunity beyond a few months or years at most. It is important to determine how long immunity lasts and, if immunity wanes, when it wanes, which would be helpful in determining whether and when booster doses are needed.

While phase 3 trials may be large, involving 10,000 or more participants, certain subgroups of the population may not have been enrolled in these studies, and it will be important to determine if those groups are at greater risk of vaccine failure than the general population and whether those groups should receive special vaccination schedules such as extra doses.

Another major issue that may not be addressed in phase 3 trials is whether the vaccine provides community or herd protection (Figure 1, page 15). Most phase 3 trials are individually randomized and assess the rates of disease in vaccinees versus placebo or comparator vaccine arms. Hence, they assess individual protection from disease induced by the vaccine. With many vaccines, individual protection against disease is also associated with protection against asymptomatic infection and with reduced shedding of the pathogen and reduced transmission to susceptible individuals. But that is not always the case. For example, the inactivated polio vaccine (IPV) prevents development of paralytic polio by preventing polioviruses from invading the central nervous system. And IPV protects the oral cavity from shedding of the virus when IPV-vaccinated persons are exposed to polioviruses, thus protecting the community from oral to oral transmission of the polioviruses. But IPV does not protect from intestinal infection. Thus, IPV recipients, if exposed to polioviruses, can shed those viruses in their stool, even though they do not develop paralytic polio. In places with poor hygiene and sanitation, such as in many countries in the developing world, IPV vaccination may protect the individual well, but not the community, as the virus can be continuously transmitted via the fecal-oral route. That is why in the developing world, OPV has been the vaccine of choice since OPV protects against shedding in the stool when a vaccinee is subsequently exposed to wild polioviruses.

Other questions that may not be answered through the phase 3 trials include the risk of causally related rare adverse events and whether there are risk factors for those adverse events that could be made contraindications for the vaccine. For example, when the oral polio vaccine (OPV) first became available in the United States in the early 1960s, there was no evidence that the vaccine could lead to polio. With experience, it was determined that very rarely, about 1 in 2 to 2.5 million doses distributed, the virus in the vaccine could actually cause polio either in the vaccinee or a close contact of the vaccinee. A risk factor for the adverse event was an underlying immune deficiency disorder. So, such disorders were made contraindications to receipt of OPV.

Vaccines can (albeit rarely) alter the immune response to the point that when the vaccinee is exposed to the natural infection, the immune system in that vaccinee makes a detrimental response in the individual instead of a protective response. This was seen, for example, with a killed (inactivated) measles vaccine, available in the United States between 1963 and 1967. The clinical syndrome, called "atypical measles," led to the withdrawal of this vaccine. Our current measles vaccine is a live attenuated or weakened virus and does not lead to "atypical measles." Rare events such as were noted with atypical measles may not be detected in the phase 3 trials. Continuing to monitor the vaccines for safety after approval helps pick up these rare events.

Most vaccines require more than one dose to induce optimal levels of protection against disease. Also, several different types of vaccines may be produced to protect against the disease. A question that arises is, for a multi-dose schedule, must you use the same vaccine for each dose of the schedule or can you "mix and match?" Usually pre-licensure studies do not include "mix and match" schedules of different vaccines. These studies, therefore, need to be addressed post-licensure.

Another question deals with whether persons with prior infection need to be vaccinated. For many diseases, such as measles, natural infection leads to permanent immunity. However, for others, such as influenza, immunity wanes, and there is a need for vaccination of persons who previously had the disease. Often, this question is not known at the time of vaccine licensure. Thus, post-licensure studies are needed to determine the duration of protective immunity in persons who had prior infection. If immunity wanes after natural infection, such persons should be vaccinated.

Systems to help monitor vaccine safety and effectiveness in the post-licensure setting

In the United States, there are several systems in place to monitor vaccine safety after vaccines are licensed and in use (Figure 2). One is the Vaccine Adverse Event Reporting System (VAERS) (see https://vaers.hhs.gov/). VAERS is a system that encourages healthcare providers, vaccinees, or parents of vaccinees to report potential safety signals called adverse events following vaccination. Adverse events include local and systemic reactions or a new illness that may be linked to the vaccine. Information is collected on the nature of the adverse event, its onset in relation to the date of vaccination, specific information on the vaccine including manufacturer, as well as other information. VAERS is most helpful in developing hypotheses regarding whether vaccines caused a clinical condition that occurred after vaccination. VAERS usually is not helpful in assessing whether the vaccine actually played a causal or coincidental role. That's because most adverse events are not specific to vaccines and are conditions or illnesses also seen in the absence of vaccination. When millions of people are vaccinated, there will be adverse events that occur after vaccination that are purely coincidental. They would have occurred anyway.

Figure 2

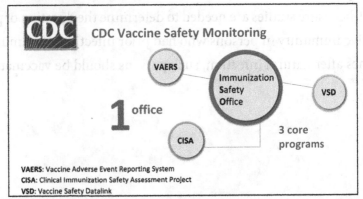

CDC Vaccine Safety Monitoring

1 office

VAERS

Immunization Safety Office

VSD

CISA

3 core programs

VAERS: Vaccine Adverse Event Reporting System
CISA: Clinical Immunization Safety Assessment Project
VSD: Vaccine Safety Datalink

An example of how VAERS works was when an initial vaccine to prevent rotavirus infection, a cause of severe infant and young child diarrhea and dehydration, was rolled out. VAERS received several clinical reports of an intestinal blockage following vaccination called "intussusception." Subsequent studies documented that this initial rotavirus vaccine was causally related with an attributable risk from vaccine of about 1 in 10,000 doses administered. This rotavirus vaccine was withdrawn from the market and subsequent large vaccine safety studies were required to show new rotavirus vaccines did not cause the intestinal blockage.

The best way to determine whether the vaccine caused the adverse event is usually to assess the occurrence (incidence rate) in vaccinees versus the incidence rate in non-vaccinees. A rate significantly higher in vaccinees would support a role for the vaccine in causing the adverse event. On the other hand, if the rates are equal, then the most likely explanation is that the adverse event was only coincidentally related. The United States has several systems in place to allow calculation of the rates of given clinical conditions in vaccinees and non-vaccinees.

The major system to evaluate causation of adverse events in the United States is the Vaccine Safety Datalink (VSD). The VSD is a collaboration between the US CDC and nine integrated healthcare organizations and has data on over 12 million persons per year. The VSD includes complete medical records in electronic databases and links vaccination records with information on healthcare visits in clinics, emergency rooms, or hospitalizations. The VSD allows calculation of rates of a given clinical condition in vaccinees versus non-vaccinees. Other ways that VSD evaluates causation is to look at the incidence rate of a given clinical condition clustered around the time of vaccination (e.g., which may be determined from VAERS reports such as the month after vaccination) versus other more distant time frames such as the month before vaccination or several months after vaccination. The FDA has a system larger than VAERS, which can perform similar studies. It is called the Post-Licensure Rapid Immunization Safety Monitoring Program (PRISM).

The VSD can also be used to monitor the effectiveness of vaccines on an ongoing basis by comparing the attack rates of a given vaccine-preventable disease in vaccinees versus non-vaccinees, in vaccinees by interval from the last vaccination, in vaccinees by the type of vaccine they received, and by the characteristics of the vaccinated and unvaccinated populations.

In addition, the CDC administers a project called the Clinical Immunization Safety Assessment Project (CISA), which includes seven participating medical centers that conduct special vaccine safety studies as well as answer complex safety questions healthcare providers raise about their patients.

The CDC also monitors vaccine effectiveness through its surveillance systems to get reports of cases of a given vaccine-preventable disease. These include networks such as the New Vaccine Surveillance Network (NVSN) (see www.cdc.gov/surveillance/nvsn/index.html). The NVSN is a population-based surveillance network that collects reports on cases of a given vaccine-preventable disease including vaccination status of those with laboratory-confirmed infections.

Another means of monitoring effectiveness is investigating outbreaks of vaccine-preventable diseases. During the investigation, the vaccination status of cases can be determined as well as the underlying vaccination status of the population in which the outbreak is occurring. Vaccination status can be assessed either from existing data on vaccine coverage in the populations, community surveys, and/or developing a set of controls in the population without illness and determining their vaccination status.

Vaccines do not save lives or reduce disease burden. Vaccinations save lives. A vaccine dose that remains in the vial is 0% effective, no matter what were the results of the clinical trial. **Vaccine hesitancy** is a reluctance or refusal to be vaccinated or to have one's children vaccinated against an infectious disease. Prior to COVID-19, vaccine hesitancy was identified by the World Health Organization as one of the top 10 global health threats of 2019. Vaccines have become victims of their own successes. Because the great majority of vaccine-preventable diseases are now rare because of vaccination, the population does not see the many diseases that vaccines prevent and hence is not fearful or does not appreciate the risk. Further, when an adverse event follows a vaccine, the adverse event is not necessarily causally related. The adverse event may be coincidental, and in fact when millions of persons are vaccinated against a given disease, coincidental adverse events following vaccination should be anticipated, since unfortunately bad things happen every day in our population unrelated to vaccination. Increased hesitancy and concern over vaccines may be stimulated by the media, particularly the social media, that reports adverse-event stories that are not supported by science.

Building and sustaining vaccine confidence is essential to achieving the benefits that vaccines can provide. For a successful campaign of vaccinations, sustaining investments not only in vaccine development but also in ways to educate and optimize the acceptance of vaccines by populations for whom the vaccines are recommended are needed. This involves investments in behavioral and communications research. To overcome vaccine hesitancy, "the right message, delivered by the right messenger, through the right communications channel" is required.

Understanding why people are hesitant and developing transparent messaging to address the concerns is critical. What is also critical is to have the message delivered by a person who is trusted by the community. Hesitant persons may trust their primary care provider, leaders in their community, someone in the clergy, people who look like them, or others. Thus, persons wanting to optimize impact of vaccines who encounter vaccine hesitancy should build collaborations with persons trusted by people with hesitancy. And it is critical to reach hesitant populations through communications channels they regularly access.

Studies of parents concerned about whether to vaccinate their children show primary care providers are a major source of trust. Further, a presumptive approach is more effective than a participatory approach. A presumptive approach is "We will give Johnny vaccines A, B, and C today. Do you have any questions?" A participatory approach would entail the following statement: "Johnny is eligible for vaccines A, B, or C today. Which if any would you like him to get?" Another effective approach has been called motivational interviewing. When a healthcare provider addresses someone who is hesitant, it is important to build trust with statements like, "I understand why you may be hesitant. It is perfectly appropriate to raise the questions about vaccines that you have raised. Let me try to answer them and then let me know if you have further questions."

There are other approaches to addressing vaccine hesitancy (see www.cdc.gov/vaccines/hcp/patient-ed/index.html and www.vaccineconfidence.org).

Chapter 3

COVID-19 Epidemiology, Virology, and Immunity

EPIDEMIOLOGY

The COVID-19 pandemic that began in Wuhan, China, in December 2019 was first reported globally on December 31, 2019, but cases likely occurred in Wuhan as early as November 2019. Several cases were associated with the bustling Wuhan Huanan Seafood Wholesale Market. The wet market (open-air stalls with vendors selling live animals, fresh seafood, meats, fruits, and vegetables) was closed December 31, 2019 and has not reopened. While no direct evidence exists that the market was the origin for the pandemic, two-thirds of the initial confirmed cases in Wuhan were linked to the location, and multiple environmental samples in the market detected SARS-CoV-2. The virus spread rapidly in Wuhan and Hubei province and was transferred via air travelers and quickly spread globally.

The first case in the United States was officially confirmed in mid-January 2020. However, based on serologic data and the genetic sequences of the virus, it appears that multiple introductions into the United States occurred in January and early February 2020 both from Asia and Europe. Early detection of COVID-19 was severely limited by the lack of availability of diagnostic testing. While the number of known cases in the United States on February 17 was 29 (after the evacuation of 14 cases from the cruise ship *Diamond Princess* in Japan), undetected cases were spreading rapidly in the country. In three waves over 2020 and into 2021, the United States by March 2021 is expected to exceed 30 million confirmed cases and 500,000 deaths. Worldwide as of the end of February 2021 there is expected to be more than 110 million cases and over 2.5 million deaths reported.

Molecular epidemiology

The COVID-19 epidemic is being tracked using the tools of molecular epidemiology. Each virus has a molecular signature or fingerprint, the genetic sequence of the virus. For SARS-CoV-2 the virus is composed of ~30,000 nucleotides. Although these are RNA viruses, the nucleotide sequence is translated into A, C, G, and T, the four building blocks of the DNA genetic code, or the complementary DNA (see below). Based on high-throughput technologies originally developed for the Human Genome Project of over 20 years ago, the genetic sequence of each virus can be rapidly determined and compared to other SARS-CoV-2 viruses. Because of mutations in the genetic code that occur at a rate estimated at approximately twenty mutations per year across the SARS-CoV-2 genome, a molecular signature is determined. Currently well over 500,000 SARS-CoV-2 isolates have been sequenced and are in databases established around the world (see www.gisaid.org/hcov19-variants/). New variants of the virus have appeared and some have become dominant globally and in specific regions. Although over 100 million cases have been documented globally, since approximately 80% of infections are asymptomatic or mildly symptomatic, the true number of undocumented infections is thus five to seven times this number.

The 2019 SARS-CoV-2 is most closely related to bat SARS-CoV-like coronaviruses. Bats likely served as a reservoir for this and other new coronaviruses. Also, there is evidence of evolution of these viruses in animals and now in human hosts. One animal, the Malayan pangolin imported into China, contains coronaviruses closely related to SARS-CoV-2 and may have served as an intermediate host for introduction of the virus.

According to the CDC, in the United States the R_0 for SARS-CoV-2 is between 2 and 4, with the best estimate thought to be 2.5.[1]) This means the average person infected with SARS-CoV-2 would infect between 2 and 4 others if they lived in a community that was 100% susceptible. However, the virus is evolving to become more infectious and transmissible. For example, the SARS-CoV-2 virus variant in the United Kingdom (which goes by the name "lineage B.1.1.7" or VUI202012/01) was shown to have an increased R_0 of 0.4. An increase of R_0 by 0.4 may sound very small, but in a 100% susceptible population, this increase adds a lot of cases. If R_0 is 2.5 in a 100%

---

1   "COVID-19 Pandemic Planning Scenarios." Centers for Disease Control and Prevention, September 10, 2020. https://www.cdc.gov/coronavirus /2019-ncov/hcp/planning-scenarios.html#five-scenarios.

susceptibility setting, the number of cases at the 10th generation of spread would equal 9,537 cases. If the R_0 is now 2.9, then the number of cases at the 10th generation is 42,071 cases. The CDC predicts the lineage B.1.1.7 variant may become the dominant virus causing COVID-19 in the United States and in other countries by March 2021. Other major variants that are emerging were first detected in South Africa, the B.1.351 variant, and Brazil, the P.1 variant. As discussed below, changes in the spike protein of the virus in these and other variants have led to increased SARS-CoV-2 infectiousness in humans as the virus has spread.

MODES OF TRANSMISSION

SARS-CoV-2 is mostly spread from person to person through respiratory droplets that travel 3–6 feet, less effectively by smaller airborne particles, and even less effectively by contact with contaminated surfaces. The amount of virus needed to cause infection is not precisely known but may be several hundred viral particles.

Figures 3a and 3b[2] (as of February 4, 2021)

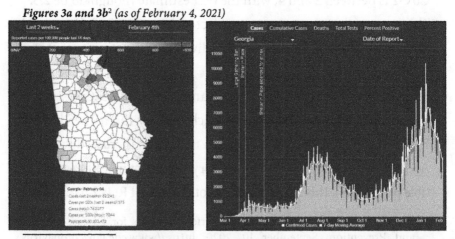

2 "COVID-19 Status Report." Georgia Department of Public Health, February 4, 2021. https://dph.georgia.gov/covid-19-daily-status-report. In converting the figure from color to black and white, some of the areas with low incidence are not showing correctly. The high incidence counties are correctly shown. Please go to the website for actual representation of all the counties.

Infected individuals both symptomatic and asymptomatic can have 10,000 to 10,000,000 viral particles per ml of nasal secretions. Although the virus can also be shed in the stool for some time after infection, there is not clear evidence that the virus is effectively transmitted by this route. Thus, masks that cover the nose and mouth, social distancing, avoiding crowds, and hand washing are the most effective control measures.

The coronavirus epidemic has occurred in multiple waves. In Figures 3a and 3b (page 48), the number of cases in Georgia are demonstrated with three distinct waves, with the third being by far the largest wave of COVID-19 cases. These waves are initiated by increased social contacts and spread (e.g., holiday gatherings), by enhanced viral infectivity (new strain variants) and are influenced by surveillance and the ability to diagnose an infection (underdiagnosis certainly was a contributor to the low magnitude of the first wave detected in March and April 2020). Infections appear to decrease and then increase in a different part of the population, resulting in the multiple waves of infection.

There are differences or "heterogeneity" in the individual transmission patterns. Superspreading events (where an individual transmits to five or more people) appear to account for 80–85% of cases, coming from just 5% of infected individuals. In cases occurring in a household setting, the secondary attack rate is 16–20% if the index case is symptomatic, less if asymptomatic. In social gatherings with friends, the secondary attack rate is 6%, travel 5%, and due to the impact of social distancing, casual close contact transmissions in the workplace are less than 2%. While both asymptomatic and symptomatic individuals can spread the virus, symptomatic individuals are three or four times more likely to be spreaders.

Public clustering of individuals can lead to the rapid spread of SARS-CoV-2. Infected individuals without or with minimal symptoms in a poorly ventilated, crowded space—particularly where people talk, shout, or sing—spread the virus. Restaurants, gyms and cafés, other gatherings (funerals, choir practice, church services, concerts, ship outbreaks, political events), account for the transmission of most COVID-19 infections in the United States. The risk of infection is proportional to the time spent in indoor public places. Ten percent of places visited account for 85% of infections. Full-service restaurants, fitness centers, cafés and snack bars, hotels and motels, limited-service restaurants, religious organizations/events, healthcare, groceries, and other stores (pet, sporting goods, general merchandise) have been linked to the highest increased transmission.

COVID-19 VIROLOGY

SARS-CoV-2 is a novel animal virus not previously known or associated with human disease. SARS-CoV-2 is a member of the **coronavirus** family named because of the crown-like spikes on the virus surface (see Figure 4, page 52). Coronaviruses are RNA viruses. That is, they are composed of a single strand of RNA (ribonucleic acid), in contrast to DNA (deoxyribonucleic acid), as the genetic material. This RNA is translated into proteins, with the nucleocapsid protein inside the virus and the surface spike protein being the most abundant. Other proteins made by the virus include nonstructural proteins (NSPs), such as NSP7 and NSP13.

The virus was named SARS-CoV-2 because of its close relationship to the coronavirus responsible for severe acute respiratory syndrome (SARS-CoV) that caused an often fatal pneumonia in a 2003 outbreak in Yunnan, Guangdong, and Hong Kong, China, with subsequent spread to Singapore, Montreal, Vietnam, Thailand and other regions. More than 70% of the genetic (i.e., nucleotide sequences—uracil, adenine, cytosine, guanine [UACG]) of SARS-CoV-2 and SARS-CoV are identical. SARS-CoV-2 also shares ~50% of its genetic sequence with the coronavirus responsible for Middle Eastern Respiratory Syndrome (MERS-CoV) identified in 2010. SARS-CoV-2 is the seventh coronavirus known to infect humans. Other human coronaviruses have been known for many years to cause the common cold with the names HCoV-229E, HCoV-NL63, HCoV-HKU1, and HCoV-OC43. The closest known relative of the SARS-CoV-2 virus is found in a species of bats (*Rhinolophus affinis*) that are found in China and Southeast Asia. Bats, as they did for SARS-CoV and MERS, serve as the reservoir host for the ancestor of SARS-CoV-2. There is likely an intermediate animal host between the bat reservoir and transmission to humans. Pangolins (*Manis javanica*) can get infected with and transmit coronaviruses related to SARS-CoV-2. For SARS-CoV, the civet cat may have functioned as an intermediate host, and for MERS it is camels that transmit the virus to humans. These new coronaviruses were likely spread to humans through a natural evolutionary process in animal reservoirs. They were not engineered in a laboratory. As we have seen repeatedly, animal viruses (Ebola, avian influenza) can jump species boundaries and are a major threat to human health.

The SARS-CoV-2 spike protein (S) is a major target for antibodies that neutralize the virus and is the basis for the vaccines that have been approved and many others in clinical trials. The spike protein binds to the human receptor angiotensin-converting enzyme 2 (hACE2) found on cells of the nose and respiratory tract to initiate infection. Since the outbreak began, there is continued evolution of the spike protein through natural mutations that more efficiently bind the human ACE receptor. This has led to increased infectivity of or prolonged shedding the virus.

Figure 4

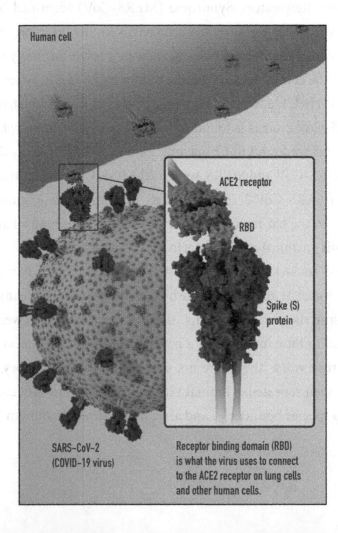

Human cell

ACE2 receptor

RBD

Spike (S) protein

SARS–CoV–2 (COVID–19 virus)

Receptor binding domain (RBD) is what the virus uses to connect to the ACE2 receptor on lung cells and other human cells.

COVID-19 IMMUNITY

The emergence of long-term (called adaptive) immunity in response to the SARS-CoV-2 virus begins within the first 7–10 days after the infection. Understanding the key features of this immunity to SARS-CoV-2 is essential in forecasting COVID-19 outcomes and for developing effective vaccines and other strategies to control the pandemic. Maintaining an immune memory against SARS-CoV-2 is also critical to understanding how long protection lasts.

Infection with SARS-CoV-2 results in most individuals in a major adaptive immune response of both the antibody-producing and cell-mediated arms of the immunity system. The antibody response is due to the robust expansion of two important immune cells, called memory B cell and plasma cells, early in infection. Two classes of these antibodies, IgM and IgA antibodies, are detected in the blood by day 5–7 and a third class, IgG, by day 7–10 after the onset of symptoms. In general, the levels of IgM and IgA antibody (measured in titers) in the blood decline after approximately 28 days, and IgG titers peak at approximately 50 days before they begin to slowly decline. Simultaneously, SARS-CoV-2 infection activates cell-mediated immune responses called T cells in the first week of infection. There are two major classes of T cells, CD4+ cells and CD8+ T cells. SARS-CoV-2 virus-specific memory CD4+ cells and CD8+ T cells peak within 2 weeks but remain detectable at lower levels for 100 or more days after infection. SARS-CoV-2–specific memory CD4+ T cells are found in up to 100% and CD8+ T cells in approximately 70% of patients recovering from COVID-19.

The magnitude or height of the antibody and T cell responses can differ among individuals and is influenced by the severity of COVID-19 (asymptomatic, mild, moderate, or severe). Higher antibody titers are often seen in individuals following more severe disease, but this may be because such individuals have large amounts of detected virus. We do not yet understand which of the immune responses correlate with protection from subsequent COVID-19 reinfection, but antibodies that neutralize the virus (neutralizing antibodies) appear critical. This is especially true of antibodies that recognize the viral receptor binding domain (RBD) and other parts of the spike (S) protein (Figures 5a and 5b) and prevent subsequent binding of the virus to the angiotensin-converting enzyme receptor. This prevents the fusion of the virus with the human cell membrane and viral entry. Thus, these neutralizing antibodies are one important potential correlate of immunity. The magnitude or number of the antibodies to SARS-CoV-2, especially the IgG antibodies to the spike protein, correlates strongly in convalescing patients with virus neutralization.

Figure 5a   *Figure 5b*

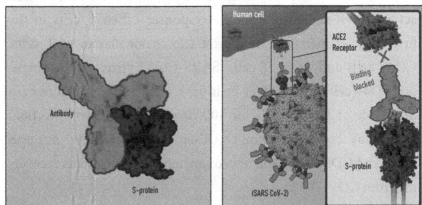

The generation of neutralizing antibodies directed at the spike protein is the basis of multiple human vaccines in clinical trials to counteract SARS-CoV-2. Virus neutralization is also the basis of single specific antibodies (called monoclonal antibodies) that have been isolated and manufactured and given to prevent or treat COVID-19 human disease. Neutralizing antibodies to SARS-CoV-2 have been shown to be protective in animal models of COVID-19 infection. Potent neutralizing antibodies and CD4$^+$ T cell responses to the spike protein protect against SARS-CoV-2 infection in the lungs and nose of studies in nonhuman primates without evidence of any adverse impact.

Recent reports have demonstrated a decline in neutralizing antibodies to SARS-CoV-2 over the months in patients recovering from infection, raising concern of susceptibility to reinfection. Antibody levels always decline after the acute phase of an infection. A similar pattern of decline is seen with T cell responses. After this reduction, antibody is maintained by the smaller number of long-lived plasma cells that reside in the bone marrow and constitutively produce and secrete antibody in the absence of antigen. When the virus is encountered again, an antibody "recall" response comes from this pool of memory B cells that are also long-lived. In fact, only a few circulating memory B cells have been shown to mature and produce highly potent neutralizing antibodies even when serum neutralizing titers are low. Thus, an early decline of neutralizing antibody levels should not be of concern. The key is the levels of antibody titers that stabilize after natural infection or vaccination and that memory B cells develop. Recent studies indicate that balanced immune memory responses including antibody, memory B cells, and T cells persist for at least eight months in COVID-19 patients who have recovered.

About one-third of patients who have recovered from COVID-19 do have initial low levels of antibodies and low viral neutralizing activity, especially among individuals who have had mild or asymptomatic disease. Given the wide range of clinical disease, this variability in the antibody responses among patients with COVID-19 is expected. As noted, the amount of virus present is a major driver of the magnitude of the response, as notably the highest amounts of neutralizing antibodies are found in individuals recovering from severe disease, but other factors also may be involved in this immune response.

Some important lessons have come from previous studies of the coronaviruses that cause the common cold. The immunity and the reinfections to the common cold coronaviruses, human coronavirus (HCoV) OC43, HCoV 229E, and HCoV HKU1, provide important lessons about our potential immune future to SARS-CoV-2. The work indicates that unlike some infections such as measles, protective immunity to coronaviruses is not lifelong. In some of these studies, humans were challenged in a controlled and isolated situation with one of the circulating common cold coronaviruses (HCoV 229E). Antibodies to the virus waned over the first year after the initial viral nasal challenge, suggesting that protection against repeated infections with common cold coronaviruses lasts only one or two years. However, after re-challenge with the same HCoV 229E strain at one year, no individuals who had previously been infected developed a cold and all had a shorter duration of detectable virus shedding. Thus, strain-specific immunity to clinical coronavirus disease may be preserved despite the rapid waning of antibodies. More than a year into the outbreak and after millions and millions of infections globally, reports of reinfection mostly after initial mild COVID-19 illness are appearing. Although a complete understanding of these individuals and their initial immune response is not yet clear, reinfection with SARS-CoV-2 suggests that the natural human immune response may not provide immunity that is completely protective, "sterilizing" immunity, but it may shorten shedding of the virus, reduce spread, and prevent severe disease. Further, at this point the number of documented reinfections is very low compared to the number of total infections, suggesting most infected persons maintain, at least for six months to a year, protective immunity. Very different strains of the virus expressing modified spike proteins are likely to increase reinfections since antibodies to the spike protein may be less effective, but a base of immunity to this virus is being created in the population. Reinfections with new variant viruses have been reported in the literature and in vaccine clinical trials.

The T cell immune arm also appears to be important in creating immunity to SARS-CoV-2 virus. SARS-CoV-2–specific memory T cells called CD4+ and CD8+ T cells are also generated in both asymptomatic and severe COVID-19. These T cells can kill SARS-CoV-2-infected cells and express antiviral proteins called cytokines, features that in addition to antibody may control viral replication and prevent recurrent severe infections. Individuals with mild or asymptomatic disease are reported to exhibit robust memory T cell responses months after COVID-19 infection. An important question that remains to be answered is whether memory T cells in the absence of detectable circulating antibodies protect against SARS-CoV-2. The identification of SARS-CoV-2–specific T cells may have future utility to assess SARS-CoV-2 exposure before antibodies arise and after their decline. At present, our understanding of T cell contributions in the prevention of severe COVID-19 is limited. Also, these T cells, if present in the lung and other tissues, may exert an antiviral protective role. Also, in contrast to antibodies to the SARS-CoV-2 spike protein that show little cross-reactivity to the seasonal coronaviruses, there is evidence of preexisting T cell immunity to SARS-CoV-2 in the blood of donors collected either prior to the COVID-19 pandemic or among those without clinical infection. These preexisting T cells likely represent responses induced by previous infection with the other human coronaviruses (see above) known to be one of the causes of the common cold. The T cells can cross-react and recognize SARS-CoV-2 expressed proteins such as the nucleocapsid (N protein) and spike structural proteins as well as the nonstructural proteins (NSPs) NSP7 and NSP13 produced by the virus. T cells reactive to SARS-CoV-2 are also seen in the household contacts of patients infected with SARS-CoV-2 but who do not have a history of COVID-19. While the RBD region of the SARS-CoV-2 spike protein shows little similarity to the seasonal coronaviruses, cross-reactive T cells from these previous "cold" coronavirus infections have been boosted with exposure to SARS-CoV-2. Do these preexisting T cells shape our immune response to SARS-CoV-2 natural exposure or following COVID-19 vaccination, as well as influence the severity of COVID-19? Overall, the scientific evidence suggests T cells are another important level of immunity against COVID-19.

Thus, in the year since recognition of COVID-19 and SARS-CoV-2, the key paths to long-term immunity against COVID-19 are being unraveled, and vaccines exploiting this knowledge have been developed and are now in expanded clinical use.

Chapter 4

Introduction to COVID-19 Vaccines

The development of vaccines directed at SARS-CoV-2 to prevent COVID-19 has been underway since the beginning days of the outbreak in early 2020. As of late January 2021, WHO (Addendum A) lists 237 vaccines in development and 63 in human clinical trials. Currently, there are 16 phase 3 COVID-19 vaccine trials globally that are enrolling or that have enrolled all needed participants. As reviewed below, these vaccines are based on several vaccine "platforms": purified protein (2), non-replicating viral vectors (4), inactivated virus (6), mRNA (3), or DNA (1). In the completed US phase 3 COVID-19 vaccine trials, individuals 16–18 years and older, including the elderly, individuals with underlying medical conditions, and from broad racial and ethnic backgrounds were enrolled. Phase 3 trials are blinded to the investigators and participants and are randomized to include vaccine and a "placebo" arm. The placebo may receive another vaccine or, in most studies, an injection of normal saline. Phase 3 trials are conducted to determine the efficacy and safety of the vaccine in a large population. Once efficacy is shown, the placebo recipients in these studies are "crossed over" to receive the vaccine.

In addition, there are over 174 COVID-19 vaccine candidates undergoing preclinical studies. These vaccines in preclinical studies include the platforms noted above as well as other novel platforms: replicating viral vectors, live attenuated virus, and replicating and non-replicating viral vectors including antigen presenting cells.

In the United States, in just over 11 months, two mRNA vaccines were developed and manufactured in parallel, tested in phase 1, 2, and the phase 3 large clinical trials, found to be safe and efficacious, and distributed initially in December 2020 to healthcare workers and residents of long-term care facilities, followed by those over 65 and with underlying medical conditions in January 2021. The story of that remarkable scientific and manufacturing accomplishment is described later in this chapter.

Why do these vaccines work? What is an immune correlate of protection? Vaccines are designed to induce a human immune response that prevents individual disease and may prevent or shorten individual infections. Much of the background for SARS-CoV-2 vaccines was initially based on the research on SARS-CoV infections, which in 2003 caused a global outbreak in 26 countries, the work on another novel coronavirus MERS, the long-term studies of other coronaviruses, and the work on other respiratory viruses such as respiratory syncytial virus (RSV).

In addition to individual protection, vaccines may also induce community or "herd" protection by decreasing transmission of the virus from one individual to another. We know that the two initial mRNA vaccines prevent illness with 94–95% efficacy in individuals. However, we do not yet know if they prevent infection or transmission.

One or two doses? While one dose of a vaccine would be ideal for control of the outbreak, for most of the COVID-19 vaccines becoming available, two doses are necessary to achieve high levels of protection against disease. Unlike weak (attenuated) live virus vaccines that control mumps, measles, and chickenpox, the current COVID-19 vaccines are not live viruses but are directed at a single protein, the SARS-CoV-2 spike protein. However, there is no intact virus or replication of the SARS-CoV-2 virus in these vaccines. While there may be some protection after the first dose, the second dose provides a boost to the immune system and magnifies the immune response to spike protein of SARS-CoV-2. As an example, the amount of antibody to the spike protein and the ability to neutralize the virus are increased a hundredfold after the second or booster dose. This level of antibody is slower to decline and prolongs protection.

MAJOR COVID-19 VACCINE TARGET: THE SARS-COV-2 SPIKE PROTEIN

The spike protein extends from the surface of the virus (Figure 6, page 67). Each of the structures shown is composed of three spike proteins (trimer) bundled together. The spike protein is the part of the virus that initially attaches to human cells. The top of the spike protein recognizes a molecule present on the surface of many kinds of human cells called the ACE2 receptor. What is an ACE2 receptor? ACE2 stands for angiotensin-converting enzyme 2 receptor. Angiotensin is a chemical that narrows your blood vessels and increases your blood pressure. Angiotensin receptor blockers (ARBs) are medications that block the action of angiotensin II by preventing angiotensin II from binding to receptors on the cells surrounding blood vessels. The ACE2 receptor is found in abundance on cells that line the back of the nose and the lung. Once the SARS-CoV-2 virus binds to the ACE2 receptor, a series of events leads to fusion of the lower portion of the spike protein and virus with the human cell membrane. Human proteins that act as enzymes, the transmembrane protease serine 2 (TMPRSS2) and the Furin protease, cleave the spike (S) protein of SARS-CoV-2. This facilitates the fusion of SARS-CoV-2 with human cellular membranes and leads to viral entry. Inside the cell, the virus replicates to high levels. The replicated virus is then shed from the cell to infect other cells or is transmitted in respiratory droplets and aerosols.

The SARS-CoV-2 spike protein is the target for the COVID-19 vaccines but must be presented to the human immune system in a way that allows a neutralizing immune response to the vaccine. In the design of most of the vaccines authorized for emergency use or in development, the spike protein is expressed as a stabilized protein prior to its fusion with human cells. In previous studies with SARS-COV and other viruses, the presentation of this structure was critical to achieve a robust virus neutralization immune response.

A lot of attention (justifiably so) has been directed to the mutations in the spike protein that have arisen during the pandemic. Most of these mutations do not persist in the populations but several of these mutations do increase the ability of the spike protein to attach to the ACE receptor on human cells, increasing infectivity or shedding of the virus and the spread of the virus. However, COVID-19 infection and the vaccines induce multiple different antibodies and T cell responses to the spike protein. Some of the recent variants (e.g., B.1.351) do decrease virus neutralization by the antibodies from convalescent COVID-19 patients and from vaccinees. One advantage of several of the vaccine platforms is that changes to the spike protein can be rapidly engineered into modifications of the vaccines. Work on such modified versions of the vaccines is underway.

One such spike mutation, D614G, emerged in early March 2020 and became the global dominant strain; this mutation, which resulted in a change in a protein building block amino acid—from aspartic acid (D) to another amino acid glycine (G) at position 614 of the protein sequence of the spike protein—is associated with higher viral loads in patients and in cell culture and animal models. The mutation increases the binding of the viral spike protein to the human ACE2 receptor and fusion with the cell, leading to enhanced virus infectivity.

Mutations leading to new variants in the SARS-CoV-2 spike protein are a concern. The "D614G" variant, which does increase infectivity, does not reduce the recognition of spike protein by neutralizing antibody. In fact, for the D614G variant, antibody binding to the spike protein is enhanced.

As noted above, the SARS-CoV-2 virus B.1.1.7 lineage variant initially identified in the United Kingdom (UK) in the fall of 2020 was associated with a rapid increase in COVID-19 cases in southeast England, leading to enhanced epidemiological and virologic investigations. Analysis of the SARS-CoV-2 viral genome identified a large proportion of these cases belonged to a new single virus cluster (e.g., lineage B.1.1.7). This variant is now rapidly spreading globally. The new variant contained multiple spike protein mutations present as well as mutations in other viral genomic regions. The variant is significantly more transmissible than previously circulating variants, with an estimated potential to increase the reproductive number (R_0) by 0.4 or greater with an estimated increased transmissibility of up to 70%. There is also some recent evidence that it might be associated with increased disease severity. However, studies indicate viral neutralization and vaccine efficacy are preserved against the B.1.1.7 variant.

As noted, recently other SARS-CoV-2 variants have emerged in South Africa (501Y.V2 or B1.351), Brazil (484K.V2 or P.1), and the United States (B.1.429), and these have been detected in other countries. These variants also contain multiple mutations in the spike protein and appear to also increase infectivity. Whether these variants increase the severity of infections is under investigation. The recent variants B.1.351 and P.1 do show decreased virus neutralization by the antibodies from convalescent COVID-19 patients and from vaccinees. However, antibodies alone may be only one correlate of protection. Current evidence indicates that the COVID-19 vaccines that may generate antibody and T cells (CD-8+ cells) being deployed retain significant efficacy against these variants, especially in the prevention of severe disease (Chapter 6). Additional studies are underway to determine if these variants impact natural or vaccine-induced immunity.

Figure 6: SARS-CoV-2 spike protein extending from virus surface

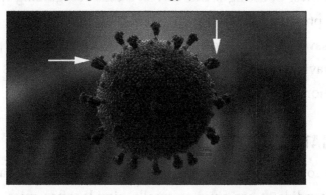

Seroprevalence data (antibodies to the SARS-CoV-2 spike protein) estimate that there may be 5–7 times more SARS-CoV-2 infections than the number of reported cases. Thus, as many as a third
(33%) of the US population to date may have been infected when
assessed by those with a detectable immune response to SARS-
CoV-2. However, relying on population-based natural immunity,
especially for populations at risk of greatest disease severity, is not
wise. Boosting specific neutralizing antibodies and T cell immunity to high levels with an effective vaccine, regardless of prior
immune status, may further protect these individuals.

COVID-19 vaccines are focused on the prevention of clinical infection, disease severity, or both. These vaccines show the
induction of a strong immune response to the spike protein, especially with a second dose that can generate high levels of neutralizing antibodies comparable with or greater than those seen in
blood samples from patients who are recovering from COVID-19.
Inclusion of vaccine boosts, employed for several other vaccines
where circulating antibody levels are critical for protection, may
be needed to maintain levels of anti–SARS-CoV-2 neutralizing

antibodies. Boosting SARS-CoV-2 T cells recognizing spike and other proteins may also be crucial in limiting replication and disease severity. SARS-CoV-2 may well follow the path of previous coronaviruses and become endemic in the population as another common cold virus.

INITIATING COVID-19 VACCINE STUDIES

Prior to the administration of vaccines to humans, early vaccine candidates are given to small animals, often mice, and the immune responses and safety of the vaccines are measured. The vaccine must generate immunity in the tested animals and not cause harm. With SARS-CoV-2, nonhuman primates have also been used in early COVID-19 vaccine studies, as outlined below.

Earlier vaccines for SARS-CoV-1 and Middle East respiratory syndrome coronavirus paved the way for rapid development of SARS-CoV-2 vaccines. Two small studies of SARS-CoV-1 vaccines in humans were completed, but work was halted once the virus was eliminated from circulation. After MERS-CoV emerged, early human vaccine studies were also conducted against this virus and demonstrated that the vaccines triggered immunity and were not associated with concerning side effects.

Immunologic basis for SARS-CoV-2 vaccination

Several studies supported the concept that vaccination had the potential to prevent SARS-CoV-2 infection. Experimental infection with wild-type SARS-CoV-2 virus in nonhuman primates who had been previously infected with COVID-19 were protected against subsequent reinfection, indicating that infection resulted in protection against another subsequent infection. In addition, vaccination of primates also protected against viral challenge. Both neutralizing antibodies and T cells (CD 8+ cells) are important in protection. Thus, it appeared that vaccines that generated neutralizing antibody and/or T cell immunity could offer protection against COVID-19.

Figure 7: Platforms for SARS-CoV-2 vaccines in development

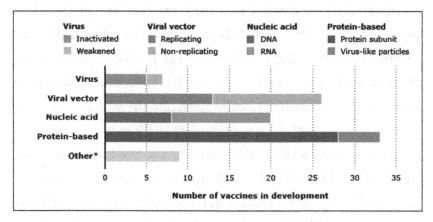

This reflects vaccines under development as of mid-2020. The World Health Organization maintains an updated list of COVID-19 vaccine candidates on their website (www.who.int/publications/m/item/draft-landscape-of-covid-19-candidate-vaccines).

SARS-CoV-2: severe acute respiratory syndrome coronavirus 2.

* Other efforts include testing whether existing vaccines against poliovirus or tuberculosis could help to fight SARS-CoV-2 by eliciting a general immune response (rather than specific adaptive immunity) or whether certain immune cells could be genetically modified to target the virus.

Vaccine platforms

SARS-CoV-2 vaccines are being developed using several different platforms. Some of these platforms use traditional approaches, such as inactivated virus or live attenuated viruses, which have been used for inactivated influenza vaccines and the measles vaccine, respectively. Other approaches employ newer platforms, such as recombinant proteins (used for human papillomavirus vaccines) and vectors (used for Ebola vaccines). Some platforms, such as RNA and DNA vaccines, have never been employed in a licensed vaccine. General descriptions of the different platforms used for SARS-CoV-2 vaccines are presented here (Figure 7).

Inactivated vaccines: Inactivated vaccines are produced by growing SARS-CoV-2 in the laboratory and then chemically inactivating the virus. The inactivated virus is then combined with alum or another adjuvant in the vaccine to stimulate immunity. Inactivated vaccines are typically given into the muscle. Their production requires high-level containment facilities to prevent spread of the infectious SARS-CoV-2 virus to the production workers. Immunity to these SARS-CoV-2 inactivated vaccines would target not only the spike protein but also other parts of the virus, since the entire killed virus is included in the vaccine. Inactivated SARS-CoV-2 vaccines are being developed in China, India, and Kazakhstan, and several are in late-stage clinical trials.

Live attenuated vaccines: Live attenuated vaccines are produced by developing genetically weakened versions of the natural virus and then infecting the recipient of the vaccine with the weakened viruses to stimulate immunity, but not cause disease. An advantage of the live vaccines is that they can be administered intranasally, as with the live attenuated influenza vaccine, which can stimulate immunity in both the upper respiratory tract and the bloodstream. However, safety concerns with live attenuated vaccines include the potential to lose their attenuation with reversion to natural virus. Several live attenuated SARS-CoV-2 vaccines are in preclinical development, but none have reached human trials.

Recombinant protein vaccines: Recombinant protein vaccines are composed of viral proteins that have been expressed in cells of various kinds, including insect and mammalian cells, yeast cells, and plant cells. These vaccines are typically administered into the muscle. Recombinant SARS-CoV-2 vaccines are in late-phase clinical trials.

Vector vaccines: These types of vaccines use viral vectors that are either unable to grow in the vaccine recipient (*Replication-incompetent vector vaccines*) or are able to grow (*Replication-competent vector vaccines*). Most *replication-incompetent vector vaccine candidates* use adenovirus vectors. However, one problem with adenovirus vector vaccines is that preexisting immunity to the vector can reduce the immunity generated to the vaccine. This can be avoided by using viral vectors that are uncommon in humans and vectors derived from animal viruses, such as a chimpanzee adenovirus (seen in the AstroZeneca vaccine). Most SARS-CoV-2 replication-incompetent viral vector vaccines are administered into the muscle. Several are in late-phase clinical trials or have released initial efficacy data. Replication-competent vectors are derived from attenuated or vaccine strains of viruses and often stimulate high levels of immunity. Among SARS-CoV-2 vaccine candidates, replication-competent vectors have been engineered to express the spike protein in attenuated measles vaccine strain vectors, influenza virus-based vectors, and several other viruses. Several replication-competent vector vaccines are in early-phase clinical trials, but development has been stopped for some candidates in this class (Merck).

DNA vaccines: DNA vaccines consist of small pieces of DNA that, when translated into protein, express the spike protein. DNA vaccines are not capable of stimulating high levels of immunity unless they are delivered by special delivery devices, called electroporators, that release a pulse of electricity so the DNA will enter the nucleus of the cell and generate proteins that stimulate an immune response.

RNA vaccines: RNA vaccines were the first vaccines for SARS-CoV-2 to be produced and represent an entirely new vaccine approach. Small pieces of mRNA surrounded by a lipid coat are administered, the RNA is translated in human cells into the target spike protein, and this stimulates immunity. These mRNA vaccines are produced completely in the laboratory and do not need to grow in any cell to be produced. However, since the technology is new, the ability to produce large quantities of RNA vaccines has not been previously tested, and some of the mRNA vaccines must be maintained at very low temperatures, complicating storage. Two of these SARS-CoV-2 RNA vaccines have been issued an EUA for use in the general population in the United States and in other countries. None of the RNA vaccines receiving EUAs in the United States have preservatives in the vaccine vials.

APPROVED VACCINES AND VACCINE CANDIDATES IN LATE-PHASE STUDIES

The first human clinical trials of SARS-CoV-2 vaccines began in March 2020, several phase 3 trials have been enrolled, and others are nearing completion of enrollment. Many of these vaccine candidates have stimulated neutralizing antibody and cellular immunity in nonhuman primates. They have demonstrated antibody immunity, which is comparable to or higher than in patients convalescing from prior SARS-CoV-2 infection. None of the early trials identified major safety concerns, but the vaccines elicited systemic adverse effects (fever, chills, headache, fatigue, myalgia, joint pains) in a proportion of participants, some of whom rated the effects severe enough to limit daily activity.

Results of phase 3 efficacy trials have been published and have shown excellent effectiveness against disease and severe disease (see also Chapter 6). The impact on transmission and the duration of the immunity will also need to be evaluated over time.

Specific vaccines are outlined below.

mRNA-1273 (Moderna): This messenger RNA (mRNA) vaccine was one of the first vaccines for SARS-CoV-2 to be produced, and it was developed and administered to humans within two months of knowledge of the SARS-CoV-2 genome. The Moderna mRNA-1273 vaccine delivers mRNA in a lipid-covered particle that triggers expression of the spike protein. It is given into the muscle in two doses 28 days apart. Vaccination in adults older than 55 years also generated immunity comparable to that seen in the younger populations. Local and generalized reactions were common, particularly after the second dose. The Moderna mRNA-1273 vaccine had 94.1% vaccine efficacy in preventing symptomatic COVID-19 at or after two weeks following the second dose. Thirty cases in the nearly 30,000 enrolled participants were severe, and all of these occurred in the placebo group. No major safety concerns were reported. An EUA was issued from the US FDA on December 18, 2020.

BNT162b2 (BioNTech and Pfizer): This mRNA vaccine is also delivered in a lipid-covered particle to express spike protein. BNT162b2 is also given intramuscularly in two doses 21 days apart. Antibody responses to the vaccine are comparable or higher than those seen in convalescent plasma from patients who had SARS-CoV-2 infection. Immune levels in participants ≥65 years old were generally lower than in younger subjects, but still comparable to titers in convalescent plasma. Systemic adverse effects were more common after the second dose. This vaccine had 95% efficacy in preventing symptomatic COVID-19 at or after day 7 following the second dose. Nine of the 10 severe cases in the nearly 40,000 vaccine recipients occurred in the placebo group. The efficacy among adults >65 years old was also over 94%. An EUA was issued from the US FDA on December 11, 2020. On December 2, 2020, BNT162b2 was approved for use in the United Kingdom and is now approved in multiple other countries

NVX-CoV2373 (Novavax): This is a recombinant protein vaccine made of spike glycoproteins and a potent adjuvant. Adjuvants are substances added to the vaccines to increase immunity. The vaccine is given in the muscle in two doses 21 days apart. As with the other vaccines, the adjuvanted vaccine stimulated levels of immunity comparable to those in convalescent plasma from patients who had been hospitalized with COVID-19. Approximately 6% of participants experienced severe generalized symptoms (mainly fatigue, headache, myalgias, and/or malaise) following the second dose. Novavax recently reported phase 3 trial results showing a vaccine efficacy against laboratory confirmed clinical COVID-19 (mild, moderate, and severe) of 89.3%.

ChAdOxnCoV-19/AZD1222 (University of Oxford, Astra-Zeneca, and the Serum Institute of India): This vaccine is based on a replication-incompetent chimpanzee adenovirus vector that expresses the spike protein. It is given into the muscle and stimulates immunity comparable to that detected in the blood of convalescent subjects with COVID-19. Fatigue, headache, and fever were relatively common after vaccine receipt and were severe in up to 8% of recipients. In a study that included older vaccine recipients (>70 years), the vaccine was better tolerated in this age-group than in younger adults and resulted in similar antibody responses after the second dose. Overall, the vaccine has been reported to have a 70.4% efficacy in preventing symptomatic COVID-19 at or after 14 days following the second dose. But there is variability depending on several different dose regimens and inter-dose intervals used. The efficacy in the dose schedule being evaluated in the pending US phase 3 trial, the "standard dose–standard dose" regimen, was 62.1% in studies completed in other countries. However, no hospitalizations or severe cases were documented in the vaccine groups. The United Kingdom and Argentina authorized the Oxford-AstraZeneca vaccine for emergency use in late December 2020, and India and Mexico authorized the vaccine for emergency use in January 2021. The EMA/EU approved the vaccine in late January 2021.

Ad26.COV2.S (Janssen/Johnson and Johnson): This vaccine is based on a replication-incompetent adenovirus 26 vector that expresses a stabilized spike protein. It is given into the muscle and is being evaluated both as a single-dose and a two-dose schedule. Early reports indicate that the vaccine stimulates high rates of neutralizing antibodies after a single-dose vaccine dose in healthy individuals 18 to 85 years old and these responses overlapped with but were slightly lower than those in convalescent plasma. The vaccine is well tolerated with fewer than 1% reporting severe systemic reactions. Baseline seroprevalence to adenovirus 26 is low in North America and Europe, but it is moderately high in sub-Saharan Africa and Southeast Asia. Preexisting antibody to adenovirus 26 will suppress the immune response to the vaccine, although most seropositive individuals have low neutralizing titers. Recently Janssen reported that a single dose of the Ad26.COV2.S vaccine was 66% effective in prevention of moderate to severe COVID-19 occurring 28 days or later after vaccination among persons 18 years of age or older. However, protection in those over 65 with medical conditions was lower at 42%. The vaccine showed efficacy against the South Africa B.1.351 variant. Overall, the single-dose vaccine was 85% effective in preventing severe disease against all variants. Further, the vaccine was 100% effective against death. An application for an EUA has been submitted to the FDA and will be reviewed in late February 2021.

Ad5-based COVID-19 vaccine (CanSino Biologics): This vaccine is based on a replication-incompetent adenovirus 5 vector that expresses the spike protein. It is given as a single intramuscular dose, and in the published trials it stimulated an immune response in healthy adults at 28 days with only mild to moderate local and generalized reactions. However, both preexisting immunity to adenovirus 5 and older age were associated with lower antibody titers following vaccination. The vaccine has been licensed in China for limited use by the military. Earlier studies of adenovirus 5 vector HIV vaccine candidates identified an increased risk of HIV acquisition among male vaccine recipients who were uncircumcised and seropositive for adenovirus 5 at baseline, but it is uncertain whether these observations are relevant for adenovirus 5 SARS-CoV-2 vaccines. The vaccine has completed a phase 3 trial in Pakistan.

Sputnik V (Gamaleya Institute): This is a vaccine developed in Russia that uses two replication-incompetent adenovirus vectors based on the spike protein. The vaccine is given into the muscle with an initial adenovirus 26 vector dose followed by an adenovirus 5 vector boosting dose 28 days later. Early reports indicate that the vaccine was associated with mild to moderate local and generalized reactions, but SARS-CoV-2 antibody and cellular immune responses were detected. The vaccine was licensed in Russia prior to completion of any efficacy trials, but recently the results of a phase 3 clinical trial were reported with a 91.6% efficacy rate. This vaccine is also in use in Argentina.

BBIBP-CorV (Sinopharm): This is an inactivated vaccine based on a SARS-CoV-2 virus isolated from a patient in China and has added aluminum hydroxide as an adjuvant. The vaccine is given intramuscularly in two doses 28 days apart. According to early reports, all recipients of two vaccine doses developed antibodies and no severe reactions were reported. China and the United Arab Emirates authorized BBIBP-CorV for emergency use in September and then fully approved the vaccine in December. Bahrain also fully approved the vaccine in December, and Egypt authorized it for emergency use in January 2021.

CoronaVac (Sinovac): This is another inactivated SARS-CoV-2 vaccine that was developed in China that also has an aluminum hydroxide adjuvant. The vaccine is given intramuscularly in two doses 28 days apart. In early reports, the vaccine appeared safe and immunogenic in healthy individuals aged 18 to 59 years. It is approved for use in Brazil, and is in phase 3 trials in Chile, Indonesia, and Turkey.

BBB152 (Bharat Biotech International Limited): Also is a whole-virus inactivated SARS-CoV-2. The vaccine is given intramuscularly in two doses 14 days apart and is in phase 3 clinical trials.

STEPS TO COVID-19 VACCINE AVAILABILITY AND DELIVERY

Establishing efficacy

Results of phase 3 trials are necessary to assess vaccine efficacy for preventing COVID-19. The US Food and Drug Administration (FDA) has provided minimal efficacy criteria for licensure of at least 50%, with the lower bound of the statistical uncertainty at 30%. Most of the trials have as an end point for efficacy of microbiologically confirmed symptomatic COVID-19 illness, and severe COVID-19 illness is also an additional end point.

Many SARS-CoV-2 phase 3 vaccine efficacy trials are enrolling 15,000 to over 30,000 individuals in each study (generally divided equally between vaccine and comparator groups), which is the estimated number necessary to sufficiently determine vaccine efficacy over a follow-up of six months. This time frame depends on the infection rate in the control group; the higher the infection rate, the less time is needed to determine vaccine efficacy. Each trial targets a defined number of detected cases, and when that number of cases has been reported, efficacy will be assessed.

Testing the study participants to determine if they have been previously infected before vaccination is not recommended, since it is not likely that it will be used in clinical practice. However, establishing vaccine safety in individuals with prior infection is important. The FDA strongly encourages that trials enroll populations that have been disproportionately affected by the COVID-19 pandemic, in particular racial and ethnic minorities.

Results from vaccine efficacy trials may be used to establish levels of antibody or cellular immunity that correlate with protection from disease, called a correlate of protection. This requires measuring antibody titers and T cells before and after vaccination and identifying a certain level of antibody or level of cellular immunity that protects against disease. If such correlates can be established, it may be possible to license vaccines based on the achievement of these antibody or cellular levels and not require each vaccine to be tested in large clinical efficacy trials. This is an issue for a vaccine not yet authorized because if there is a correlate, such as an antibody level, you don't have to wait to see the incidence of disease in vaccine versus placebo recipients. All you need to measure is the proportion of vaccinees who achieve the correlate to allow you to estimate efficacy.

Vaccine manufacturing and storage

Given the constrained time line for testing and the need for rapid deployment of the SARS-CoV-2 vaccines, several vaccine producers started commercial production prior to the availability of phase 3 trial efficacy data so that the vaccine could be quickly made available for use as soon as it was approved. This is unusual, since vaccine production facilities for widespread use of vaccines are typically not developed until after vaccine efficacy has been established, to minimize financial risk. For SARS-CoV-2 vaccines, manufacturing capabilities have been enhanced by the issuance of government funds. As an example, the US government agreed to finance production of hundreds of millions of doses of promising vaccine candidates prior to completion of the phase 3 trials, reducing the risk for the manufacturers if the vaccines did not meet licensure criteria.

Technical requirements for storage and handling of the vaccine also pose operational challenges for widespread distribution of SARS-CoV-2 vaccine candidates. As an example, some mRNA vaccines require ultracold storage in specialized freezers. The need for vials used to hold the vaccines may also pose supply-chain issues (see the Appendix for more details).

Key issues for vaccination policies

Once a SARS-CoV-2 vaccine is authorized for use in the United States, it has to be determined who should receive priority for the vaccine and who should not and how the vaccination program would be implemented. Several expert organizations have released guidance documents for vaccine allocation approaches that maximize the individual and societal benefits of vaccination. The ACIP of the United States CDC (Chapter 2), a body that makes formal recommendations for vaccine administration, has considered an allocation framework with the primary goals of maximizing the reduction in death and serious disease, preserving societal function, reducing the burden of disease among those already facing disparities, and improving health and well-being. ACIP has recommended that the very first vaccine supplies be allocated to healthcare personnel and long-term care facility residents; these populations account for approximately 24 million individuals in the United States. Other groups that were prioritized for subsequent phases of vaccine distribution were workers in essential and critical industries, individuals at high risk for severe COVID-19 due to underlying medical conditions, and individuals 65 years and older.

The National Academies of Sciences, Engineering, and Medicine (NASEM) also proposed a four-phase allocation framework based on the ethical principles of maximum benefit, equal concern, and health inequity mitigation and on the procedural principles of fairness, transparency, and being evidence-based. The NASEM prioritized vaccination according to risks of acquiring infection, severe morbidity and mortality, negative societal impact (e.g., if essential critical societal functions depend on an individual or groups of individuals), and transmission to others. The document suggests that initial vaccine supplies be allocated to individuals with the highest risks across these categories (i.e., high-risk frontline healthcare workers, first responders, those with comorbidities highly associated with severe COVID-19, and older individuals in congregate settings). As vaccination capacity expands, allocation would be broadened to populations with progressively lower risk. They also developed a vaccine allocation tool to assess how many vaccine doses would be needed per state for each priority population within this allocation framework.

Both frameworks acknowledge that in the United States and elsewhere, certain minority populations, including Black, Latino, and Indigenous populations, have been disproportionately impacted by the pandemic because of structural inequities and social determinants of health. They emphasize that, within each risk group, equitable vaccine allocation to these and other vulnerable populations should be a priority. Finally, the World Health Organization (WHO) has proposed a framework that considers global equity concerns, including assurance of vaccine access to low- and middle-income countries.

Systems need to be in place to provide access to vaccines, and barriers to access, such as cost, need to be removed. Ongoing monitoring of vaccine effectiveness and safety is critical for evaluating issues such as waning immunity, risk for vaccine failure, and vaccine-related adverse events, particularly rare events that were not detected in pre-licensure trials. Estimations of the burden of causally vaccine-related adverse events can then be weighed against the benefits of the vaccine to determine if any changes in recommendations are warranted. Disease surveillance is crucial to determine who continues to get disease, risk factors for that disease, and the role of vaccine failure versus failure to vaccinate in disease occurrence.

Vaccine Distribution: In the United States, SARS-CoV-2 vaccines will be free of charge for any individual for whom the ACIP recommends vaccination. Vaccine providers will receive administration costs reimbursed by public or private insurers, or for uninsured patients, by the Health Resources and Services Administration's Provider Relief Fund.

ADDRESSING SPECIAL POPULATIONS

Children: Vaccine licensure will only include children once the safety and immunogenicity of the vaccine has been studied in them. Such studies are underway in older children and are planned in younger children. COVID-19 is generally less severe in children than adults; nevertheless, the risk of the MIS-C following acute infection, the risk of severe disease in children with underlying medical conditions, and the general desire to prevent COVID-19 in children remain compelling reasons for vaccine studies in children. Most vaccines for children are delivered by private healthcare providers, although many are purchased using federal or other government funds. The Vaccines for Children (VFC) program is an entitlement program for all ACIP-approved vaccines for eligible children through 18 years of age. Eligible children include those on Medicaid, those who are completely uninsured, and American Indian/Alaskan Natives. Approximately 50% of children are covered by the VFC. In addition, federal grants to states can be used to purchase vaccines to cover other children. Since SARS-CoV-2 vaccines will be free to all persons for whom the vaccines are recommended, these funding mechanisms may be used with the SARS-CoV-2 vaccines that are licensed for use in children in addition to other funding sources.

Pregnant women: Vaccine studies are also planned in pregnant women, with data and safety monitoring boards that include obstetricians experienced in vaccine studies. However, many pregnant women are currently receiving vaccines approved under the EUA.

Chapter 5

COVID-19 Vaccine Safety

A ssessing and monitoring vaccine safety is a critical part of any vaccine program. Assessment of vaccine safety begins in phase 1–3 clinical trials, and there are well-established criteria and monitoring systems in place to access local reactions and systemic reactions to vaccine candidates. Safety is a major criterion reviewed by the manufacturer, and the FDA and its external advisory committee (VRBPAC) leading to licensure. In addition, post-marketing vaccine safety assessment after issuance of an EUA or licensure of a vaccine by the FDA is mandated as part of the regulatory process. Based on signals seen in the clinical trials, FDA issues specific recommendations on what the manufacturer of the vaccine should monitor, and the manufacturer prepares a comprehensive plan to address these issues. In addition, the CDC serves a critical role in the evaluation of all vaccines and is involved in evaluating ongoing COVID-19 vaccine safety. The CDC states on its website that it has "a commitment to ensure that public health officials, healthcare providers, and the public have accurate and timely information on the safety of COVID-19 vaccines."

The period after EUA or licensure is often labeled phase 4, where post-licensure safety monitoring and research begins after a vaccine is licensed and recommended for public use. The ACIP continues to monitor vaccine safety and effectiveness data even after the vaccine's routine use and may change or update recommendations based on those data. Also, the FDA requires all manufacturers to submit samples from each vaccine lot prior to its release. Manufacturers must provide the FDA with their test results for vaccine safety, potency, and purity. Each lot must be tested, because vaccines are sensitive to environmental factors like temperature and can be contaminated during production. The FDA rarely has recalled vaccine lots, but it has happened for concerns such as mislabeling, contamination during production, and potential manufacturing problems at a production plant.

While clinical trials provide important information on vaccine safety, the data are somewhat limited because of the relatively small number (hundreds to thousands) of study participants. Rare side effects and delayed reactions might not be evident until the vaccine is administered to millions of people. In the United States, there are several systems to assess safety in the post-licensure setting; some of them are passive and rely on providers, parents, and patients to report adverse events after immunization. Others are active systems where large databases with information about vaccine administration and healthcare encounters are surveyed for adverse events or specific studies are conducted to identify those events.

In 1990, the federal government established the **Vaccine Adverse Event Reporting System (VAERS),** a surveillance system to monitor adverse events following vaccination. VAERS is a passive surveillance system where providers, parents, and patients report adverse events. If any health problem happens after vaccination, anyone—doctors, nurses, vaccine manufacturers, and any member of the general public—can submit a report to VAERS. VAERS is intended to raise questions about whether receipt of a vaccine could cause the adverse event. It does not establish that the vaccine caused the adverse event. It is used to detect possible safety problems, called signals, that may be related to vaccination. If a vaccine safety signal is identified through VAERS, scientists often conduct further studies to find out if the signal represents an actual risk. The main goals of VAERS are to:

- Detect new, unusual, or rare adverse events that happen after vaccination
- Monitor increases in known side effects, like arm soreness where a shot was given
- Identify potential patient risk factors for particular types of health problems related to vaccines
- Assess the safety of newly licensed vaccines
- Watch for unexpected or unusual patterns in adverse event reports
- Serve as a monitoring system in public health emergencies

While very important in monitoring vaccine safety, VAERS reports alone usually cannot be used to determine if a vaccine caused or contributed to an adverse event or illness. The reports may contain information that is incomplete, inaccurate, coincidental, or unverifiable. Most reports to VAERS are voluntary, which means they are subject to biases. This creates specific limitations on how the data can be used scientifically. Data from VAERS reports should always be interpreted with these limitations in mind.

The strengths of VAERS are that it is national in scope and can quickly provide an early warning of a safety problem with a vaccine. Key considerations and limitations of VAERS data:

- Vaccine providers are encouraged to report any clinically significant health problem following vaccination to VAERS, whether or not they believe the vaccine was the cause.
- Reports may include incomplete, inaccurate, coincidental, and unverified information.
- The number of reports alone cannot be interpreted or used to reach conclusions about the existence, severity, frequency, or rates of problems associated with vaccines.
- VAERS data are limited to vaccine adverse event reports received between 1990 and the most recent date for which data are available.
- VAERS data do not represent all known safety information for a vaccine and should be interpreted in the context of other scientific information.

The Vaccine Safety Datalink (VSD) is a collaborative project between the United States CDC's Immunization Safety Office and nine managed healthcare organizations to actively monitor the safety of vaccines and to conduct studies about rare and serious postvaccination adverse events. It was also established in 1990 and continues to monitor safety of vaccines and conduct studies about rare and serious adverse events following immunization. The VSD uses electronic health data from each participating site. This includes information on the types of vaccines given to each patient, the date of vaccination, and other vaccinations also administered on the same day. The VSD also uses information on medical illnesses that have been diagnosed at doctors' offices, urgent care visits, emergency department visits, and hospital stays. The VSD conducts vaccine safety studies based on questions or concerns raised from the medical literature and reports to VAERS. When there are new vaccines that have been recommended for use in the United States or if there are changes in how a vaccine is recommended, the VSD will monitor the safety of these vaccines. Since 1990, investigators from the VSD have published many studies to address vaccine safety concerns.

The **Clinical Immunization Safety Assessment project (CISA)** is a national network of vaccine safety experts from the CDC's Immunization Safety Office, seven academic medical research centers, and subject matter experts at these academic centers. Established in 2001, it provides a comprehensive vaccine safety public health service to the nation. Providers who have questions about patients with adverse events after vaccination can reach out to CISA for help in evaluating reactions. Guidance is provided regarding subsequent vaccinations, additional diagnostic tests that might be performed to evaluate the adverse event, and whether causation of the event and the vaccine can be determined.

Healthcare providers or health departments in the United States can request a consultation from CISA COVIDvax for a complex COVID-19 vaccine safety question that is (1) about an individual patient residing in the United States or vaccine safety issue and (2) not readily addressed by CDC or the ACIP.

V-SAFE is a new smartphone-based health checker for people who have received a SARS-CoV-2 vaccine. The CDC will send text messages and web-based surveys to vaccine recipients through V-SAFE to check in regarding health problems following vaccination. The system will also provide telephone follow-up to anyone who reports clinically significant adverse events. One particularly appealing aspect of this system is that it will note whether the vaccine recipient is pregnant or not and will monitor the outcome of the pregnancy.

Additional vaccine safety systems implemented for SARS-CoV-2 vaccines

Similar to systems established during the 2009 H1N1 influenza pandemic, there are several systems coordinated through the CDC that enlist multiple other healthcare groups to provide ongoing data on vaccine safety.

National Healthcare Safety Network sites: A monitoring system for vaccine safety in healthcare workers and long-term care facility residents has been established and will submit adverse events reports after COVID-19 vaccines to VAERS.

FDA Monitoring of large insurer/payer databases: A system of administrative and claims-based data has been established by the FDA to monitor vaccine safety. This includes a claims-based system within the Centers for Medicare and Medicaid Services. It also includes a system of electronic health records, administrative, and claims-based data for active surveillance and research called Sentinel.

Department of Defense VAERS: Adverse events in the DOD populations are reported to VAERS. The DOD also has a Vaccine Adverse Event Clinical System that is used for case tracking and evaluation of adverse events following immunization in DOD and DOD-affiliated populations. There is also a DOD Electronic Health Record and Defense Medical Surveillance System that monitors vaccine safety.

The Department of Veterans Affairs also has a VA Adverse Drug Event Reporting System that reports adverse events following receipt of drugs and immunizations. There is also a VA Electronic Health Record and Active Surveillance System that provides additional information on safety.

Indian Health Service (IHS): there is spontaneous adverse event reporting to VAERS for populations served by IHS and tribal facilities

Each of these safety systems has been reporting adverse events to the VAERS system, and these events have been subsequently reviewed and assessed. In the process of safety evaluation, there has been a signal detected for anaphylaxis associated with the mRNA vaccines. Anaphylaxis is a severe, potentially life-threatening allergic reaction that usually occurs within seconds or minutes of exposure to something to which you are allergic. Peanuts and bee stings are examples of exposures associated with anaphylaxis. The anaphylaxis events after the mRNA vaccines have been occurring within 15 minutes of vaccine receipt in 70% of the vaccinees and within 30 minutes in 90% of the vaccinees among vaccinees who developed anaphylaxis. Most of those suffering the reactions are women who have had a previous experience with allergic reactions, including previous episodes of anaphylaxis. Providers are aware of this complication, and all of those suffering the reactions to date have been managed promptly and successfully with the administration of epinephrine. It is projected that these events occur at a frequency of 5 in 1 million vaccine recipients of the Pfizer vaccine and in 2.5 in 1 million vaccine recipients of the Moderna vaccine. The cause of these reactions is not understood at this time. Individuals who have had this type of reaction are instructed not to receive subsequent doses of the mRNA vaccine and to see an allergist to assess potential triggers for this reaction. See Chapter 7, on contraindications to vaccination, and which gives more detail on anaphylaxis.

Chapter 6

COVID-19 Vaccines Efficacy and Effectiveness

Vaccine efficacy (VE) is calculated as the proportionate reduction in illness among vaccinees compared to illness in non-vaccinees. VE is measured by the formula: VE (%) = ((ARU−ARV)/ARU)) × 100, where ARU is the attack rate or the incidence rate in the unvaccinated and ARV is the attack rate or incidence rate in the vaccinees. For example, a 95% effective vaccine means that 19 of 20 people who are vaccinated are protected against disease. One of 20 vaccinated people is not protected.

Although the words efficacy and effectiveness are often used interchangeably, most vaccine researchers use the term "efficacy" when measuring VE obtained through phase 3 randomized controlled prospective trials. In these studies, the controls either receive the placebo or a comparator product that does not protect against COVID-19. In contrast, "effectiveness" is usually used when measuring vaccine impact through observational studies, often after vaccine approval, looking retrospectively at the incidence of disease in vaccinees versus non-vaccinees who obtained or did not obtain vaccination based on demand and availability.

When assessing VE, one can measure the impact of vaccination on the prevention of clinical disease, prevention of severe disease, and prevention of infection whether symptomatic or non-symptomatic based on the specific definitions used for each category. Measurement against the different defined outcomes can be helpful in setting policies for vaccine use. For example, COVID-19 vaccines may prevent symptomatic disease in 19 of 20 people but may not eliminate asymptomatic infection in these individuals, though they may abbreviate or shorten the course of these asymptomatic infections. Below the vaccine efficacy of the two vaccines currently authorized for emergency use in the United States is reviewed.

PFIZER-BIONTECH VACCINE

The efficacy of the Pfizer-BioNTech mRNA vaccine was measured in a large placebo-controlled phase 3 trial including 43,548 persons 16 years of age or older at 152 sites worldwide (United States, 130 sites; Argentina, 1; Brazil, 2; South Africa, 4; Germany, 6; and Turkey, 9). A total of 43,448 participants received injections: 21,720 received the vaccine and 21,728 received the placebo. Two doses of the vaccine were administered 21 days apart. The primary end point of the trial was COVID-19 defined as illness in individuals who had one of the following conditions: fever, new or increased cough, new or increased shortness of breath, chills, new or increased muscle pain, new loss of taste or smell, sore throat, diarrhea, or vomiting, and a respiratory specimen obtained during the symptomatic period (four days before or after) that was positive for the SARS-CoV-2 virus in the central laboratory.

Among 36,523 participants, 16 years of age or older, who had no evidence of prior SARS-CoV-2 infection by absence of antibody to COVID-19, eight cases of COVID-19 illness with onset at least seven days after the second dose were observed among vaccine recipients and 162 cases among the placebo recipients resulting in a **vaccine efficacy of 95.0%**. The precision of the estimate is given by something called the 95% confidence interval. This interval means that if there were 100 studies done, there is a 95% chance that the efficacy would be within these 95% confidence intervals. The confidence interval was determined to be 90.3–97.6% for the Pfizer-BioNTech Vaccine; that is, we can expect with a high degree of confidence to see 90.3–97.6%. efficacy of this vaccine in the population. Among adults ≥65 years who had other medical comorbidities or obesity, the Pfizer-BioNTech vaccine efficacy was determined to be 91.7% (95% CI 44.2-99.8). The smaller number of those enrolled who were ≥65 years contributes to the wider confidence intervals.

The efficacy against severe COVID-19 was also evaluated. Severe disease was defined as having clinical signs at rest that are indicative of severe systemic illness with COVID-19; respiratory failure; evidence of shock; significant acute kidney, liver, or neurologic dysfunction; admission to an intensive care unit; or death. There were 10 cases of severe disease in the phase 3 study; nine had received the placebo and one had been vaccinated.

Among the entire trial population, the rate of COVID-19 in the Pfizer-BioNTech mRNA vaccine group started to decrease, compared to the rate in the placebo group, approximately two weeks after the first dose. This suggests initial efficacy of a single dose (the estimated vaccine efficacy of the single dose was 52% in the time before the second dose, and the 95% CI was 29.5–68.4% between the two doses). However, the actual magnitude and duration of protection from a single dose is unknown because most participants received the second dose three weeks after the first. The high efficacy was similar by gender, race, ethnicity, and underlying clinical conditions.

MODERNA MRNA 1273 VACCINE

The Moderna mRNA vaccine was tested in a large placebo-controlled phase 3 trial involving two doses of vaccine administered at a 28-day interval. The primary end point was also clinical disease and the clinical criteria for COVID-19 in participants included laboratory-confirmed SARS-CoV-2 infection and at least two of the following symptoms: fever (temperature ≥100.4 F), chills, muscle aches, headache, sore throat, or new smell or taste disorder, or at least one respiratory sign or symptom (including cough, shortness of breath, or clinical or X-ray evidence of pneumonia) and a positive laboratory test for the virus. Severe COVID-19 was defined as: respiratory rate of 30 or more breaths per minute; heart rate at or exceeding 125 beats per minute; an oxygen saturation at 93% or less while the participant was breathing room air; respiratory failure; acute respiratory distress syndrome; evidence of shock (low systolic blood pressure <90 mm Hg or diastolic blood pressure <60 mm Hg, or a need for drugs to raise the blood pressure); clinically significant acute kidney, liver, or neurologic dysfunction; admission to an intensive care unit; or death.

Of the original 30,420 participants randomized in the trial, 29,148 were eligible for analysis, including 14,548 who received placebo and 14,550 who received the mRNA 1273 vaccine. There were 269 cases of clinical COVID-19 in the placebo recipients and 19 in the vaccine recipients. The vaccine efficacy against clinical COVID-19 14 or more days after dose 2 in adults 18 years of age or older was **94.1%** with the 95% confidence interval of 89.3–96.8%. The efficacy was highest in adults 18–64 years (95.6% with 95% CI 90.6–97.9%) and slightly lower in adults 65 years of age and older (86.4% with a 95% CI of 61.4–95.2%) Thirty cases were defined as severe, and all of these cases occurred in the placebo group. Among approximately 2,000 participants who only received a single dose of vaccine or placebo, vaccine efficacy following the first dose was 80.2% (95% CI 55.2–92.5); however, these individuals only had a median follow-up time of 28 days, so the duration of protection from a single dose remains uncertain. A preliminary analysis also suggested a reduction in asymptomatic infections between dose 1 and 2. The high efficacy was similar by gender, race, ethnicity, and underlying clinical conditions.

Further information on the status of COVID-19 vaccines can be found at the following World Health Organization (WHO) Website: www.who.int/publications/m/item/draft-landscape-of-covid-19-candidate-vaccines. As of February 14, 2021, 66 vaccines were in clinical trials and an additional 176 vaccines were in preclinical development.

ASTRAZENICA CHIMP ADENOVIRUS COVID-19 VACCINE (CHADOX2 COVID-19 VACCINE)

While this vaccine has not been authorized for emergency use in the United States as of the end of January 2021, phase 3 trials have been completed in other countries, and a phase 3 trial has completed enrollment in the United States. The vaccine has been approved by the EMA (January 29, 2021). This section describes the efficacy results in randomized controlled trials in the United Kingdom, Brazil, and South Africa.

The vaccine was tested in a two-dose schedule, administered intramuscularly 28 days apart. Most of the trial participants received two standard doses of vaccine, 5×10^{10} viral particles per dose (Standard Dose, SD). A subset of participants received a half dose (Low Dose, LD) as their first dose followed by a standard dose (SD) as the second dose. Instead of a placebo, the comparator arm consisted of persons who received a meningococcal conjugate vaccine, MenACWY. The primary outcome measure was virologically confirmed COVID-19 associated with at least one of the following symptoms or signs (fever >= 37.8 C, cough, shortness of breath, and/or loss of the sense of smell or taste).

The vaccine efficacy overall was 70.4% (95% CI 54.8–80.6%). Among recipients of the LD/SD regimen, the efficacy was 90.0% (95% CI 67.4–97.0%). Among recipients of the SD/SD regimen, the efficacy was 62.1% (95% CI 41.0–75.7%). The vaccine efficacy was higher in persons who received their second dose six or more weeks after the first dose (65.4% 95% CI -2.5-78.8%) compared to those who received the second dose less than six weeks after the first dose (53.4% 95% CI 41.1-79.6%). The efficacy was much higher against clinical disease than among persons with asymptomatic infections or whose clinical symptoms, if any, were unknown (58.3% versus 7.8%). This suggests the vaccine was more effective at protecting against clinical illness than asymptomatic infection. In individuals who received two doses of the vaccine, they were 54% less likely to have an infection confirmed by NP swab, regardless of whether they had symptoms. However, the information is not adequate to determine if the vaccine did or did not reduce transmission. The efficacy of the vaccine in the UK was similar for the now dominant B.1.1.7 variant but has proven substantially less effective for the B.1.351 South Africa variant.[1]

NOVAVAX VACCINE (NVX-COV2373 RECOMBINANT PROTEIN COVID-19 VACCINE)

On January 28, 2021, Novavax made public in a press release the preliminary results regarding vaccine efficacy from their clinical trials in the United Kingdom and South Africa.[2] In the United Kingdom, the trial enrolled more than 15,000 participants between 18 and 84 years of age. Of those participants, 27% were over 65 years of age. The interim analysis was based on 62 cases, 56 in the placebo group and six cases in the vaccine group. This resulted in a vaccine efficacy against laboratory confirmed clinical COVID-19 (mild, moderate, and severe) of 89.3% (95% CI 75.2-95.4%). Of the 62 cases, only one was severe, a case in the placebo group. They

---

1   "Safety and efficacy of the ChAdOx1 nCoV-19 (AZD1222) Covid-19 vaccine against the B.1.351 variant in South Africa." Medrxiv.org, February 12, 2021. www.medrxiv.org/content/10.1101/2021.02.10.21251247v1.full.pdf.

2   "Novavax COVID-19 Vaccine Demonstrates 89.3% Efficacy in UK Phase 3 Trial." Novavax Inc. - IR Site, January 28, 2021. https://ir.novavax.com/news -releases/news-release-details/novavax-covid-19-vaccine-demonstrates -893-efficacy-uk-phase-3.

were able to evaluate the efficacy both against the previously dominant strain of SARS-CoV-2, upon which the vaccine was based,
as well as the variant B.1.1.7 circulating in the United Kingdom.
Overall, the efficacy against the older strain was 95.6% and against
the UK variant was 85.6%. The confidence intervals around these
estimates were not provided in the press release.

The vaccine efficacy from South Africa was calculated based
on data from a phase 2 study in that country, which enrolled
4,400 persons (data were not yet available from a larger phase 3
trial). Of persons who were not infected with the AIDS virus, the
efficacy was 60% (95% CI 19.9-80.1%) for prevention of symptomatic COVID-19. This was based on 29 cases in the placebo group
and 15 in the vaccine group. Only one case was severe, a case
in the placebo group, but the population enrolled was younger.
Importantly, preliminary information on the SARS-CoV-2 strains
was available on 27 of 44 infections. Of these, 92.6% (25 of 27) rep-
resented the rapidly emerging B.1.351 variant, the "South African"
variant, for which concern has been expressed regarding whether
COVID-19 vaccines based on older strains will confer protection
against new variant strains. The implications of the 60% estimate
are that significant but reduced protection was provided against
this variant.

JOHNSON & JOHNSON VACCINE (AD26.COV2.S COVID-19 VACCINE)

On January 29, 2021, Johnson & Johnson released preliminary
results of a phase 3 single-dose vaccine efficacy trial.[3] The efficacy

---

3 "Johnson & Johnson." Content Lab U.S., January 29, 2021. https://www.jnj
   .com/johnson-johnson-announces-single-shot-janssen-covid-19-vaccine
   -candidate-met-primary-endpoints-in-interim-analysis-of-its-phase-3
   -ensemble-trial.

data were based on 44,325 vaccine trial participants who received a single dose, among whom 468 cases of COVID-19 occurred. The single-dose vaccine was 66% effective in prevention of moderate to severe COVID-19 occurring 28 days or later after vaccination among persons 18 years of age or older. Overall, the single-dose efficacy was 85% effective in preventing severe disease. Further, the vaccine was 100% effective against hospitalization and death. Severe disease was defined as: hospitalization, admission to an intensive care unit, need for mechanical ventilation, and death. Moderate disease was defined as: evidence of lower respiratory tract disease (e.g., pneumonia), clots in the deep veins, shortness of breath, and clinical measurements including abnormal blood oxygen levels or two or more symptoms suggestive of COVID-19.

While no data were provided in the press release, the statement said that protection was consistent across race, age-groups, including those >60 years of age, and across variants in the group enrolled in South Africa. About 95% of the cases of COVID-19 in South Africa were the variant SARS-CoV-2 B.1.351. Data from the two-dose administration are not yet available.

WHAT IS STILL UNKNOWN ABOUT THE EFFICACY OF THE NEW COVID-19 VACCINES?

The randomized placebo-controlled trials present clear evidence that multiple COVID-19 vaccines using different platforms are highly effective against clinical COVID-19 and especially effective in preventing severe disease. What is not as clear is the duration of immunity since follow-up of individuals in the data presented from clinical trials or for EUA was only a few weeks or months after completion of the vaccination series. Also unclear is the effectiveness against asymptomatic infection and most importantly against transmission. Many available vaccines against other viruses and bacteria do prevent not only disease but also transmission. But there are some exceptions. For example, the inactivated polio vaccine (IPV) is highly effective in preventing viral invasion of the central nervous system and paralysis. But it does not prevent intestinal infection with the virus well. Thus, persons can be infected silently, shed virus in their stool, and where hygiene and sanitation are poor, infect others with the virus. It is likely the COVID-19 vaccines will decrease viral load and shedding even in asymptomatic individuals, but whether COVID-19 vaccines will completely prevent transmission remains to be determined.

Also to be determined is whether there are risk factors for vaccine failures, which could lead to alternative schedules for such persons, such as extra booster doses. Similarly, with the emergence of variants of SARS-CoV-2 viruses, it is not currently clear whether the vaccines will be as effective against some of these variants as they were against the SARS-CoV-2 virus which circulated when the vaccines were tested. If effectiveness is reduced, new or modified vaccines may be needed to deal with the variants. The induction of immunity to influenza could be a model for the induction of immunity to SARS-CoV-2. Influenza viruses mutate frequently and thereby overcome the immunity induced by prior infections or by vaccination. That is why influenza vaccines are updated annually based on strains of the virus predicted to circulate in the upcoming season. While the SARS-CoV-2 mutation rate was initially thought to be lower than influenza, variants in the spike protein are emerging and updated or second generation vaccines may well be needed to enhance protection against COVID-19 in the future.

All of this highlights the important need to have surveillance systems in place to monitor COVID-19 vaccine effectiveness on an ongoing basis. In the United States, many of the existing surveillance systems that have been established by the CDC to monitor the burden of influenza and the impact of vaccine on this burden are going to be used to measure the impact of vaccine on COVID-19. These surveillance systems can use a variety of study designs to assess vaccine effectiveness. Study designs include population-based studies in which vaccination status is determined. Surveillance systems detect COVID-19 cases and determine the vaccination status of the infected. This allows calculation of the attack rates in vaccinees and non-vaccinees leading to an estimate of the vaccine effectiveness. Another type of study is called a case-control study. Cases of COVID-19 are identified, and their vaccination status determined. Then controls are selected from well individuals who have similar characteristics as the cases, such as age, gender, and location of residence, as well as other characteristics, and their vaccination status is determined. The proportion of persons vaccinated among the cases versus controls allows estimation of the vaccine effectiveness.

A variant of the case-control study is called the "test-negative" study design. In this type of study, the cases are persons who seek medical care for an illness compatible with COVID-19 and test positive for SARS-CoV-2. The controls are persons who test negative. The vaccination status of each group is determined, which allows calculation of the vaccine effectiveness. An advantage of the test-negative design is that it minimizes bias that may occur with other studies regarding seeking of medical care. For example, vaccinated people may be more likely to seek medical care than unvaccinated people. Thus, in a traditional case-control study, there may be a bias toward a high proportion of cases among vaccinees leading to a falsely low vaccine effectiveness. In contrast, because in a test-negative design all cases and controls have sought medical care, this bias is minimized.

Community protection can be evaluated in a variety of fashions. One of the most common ways is to measure the vaccine coverage in different communities and determine whether the reduction in COVID-19 cases exceeds that based on what would be predicted. Community evaluation is based only on vaccine coverage rates and the predicted induction of population immunity.

Chapter 7

COVID-19 Vaccine Recommendations, Access, and Distribution

ALLOCATION

Eventually, COVID-19 vaccines are likely to be recommended for all populations for whom the vaccines have been demonstrated to be both safe and effective. However, until vaccine supplies are available to provide the number of doses needed to vaccinate such large populations, there is a need to prioritize the use of the vaccines. In considering priorities for COVID-19 vaccines, several factors are weighed, including how to protect those most vulnerable to complications from COVID-19 and the need to ensure essential services needed for society to function are maintained.

In the United States, the ACIP (Chapter 2), which advises the CDC, has played a major role in establishing priorities for COVID-19 vaccines. Such guidance is considered at the state level and could be modified by states. The ACIP has adopted two phases and within phase 1 has recommended three subphases (1a, 1b, and 1c). Phase 1a consists of healthcare personnel (HCP) and residents and staff of long-term care facilities (LTCF). At the time the ACIP made its recommendations for phase 1a, data available to the committee showed that as of December 1, 2020, there had been approximately 245,000 cases of COVID-19 and 858 deaths reported in HCP. The reasons for putting HCP in the highest-priority group is twofold. First, HCP are at greater risk of infection than the general population since they are involved with taking care of COVID-19 cases and hence can be frequently exposed to the virus. Second, it is critical that the infrastructure that provides care for COVID-19 patients is maintained, not only to care for COVID-19 patients but also for all of the other illnesses and conditions that require care from HCP.

LTCF are defined as facilities that provide medical and personal care, as well as other services, to persons who cannot live independently. Data considered by the ACIP, as of November 15, 2020, estimated that about 500,000 cases of COVID-19 resulting in approximately 70,000 deaths had been reported among residents of skilled nursing facilities, a subset of LTCF. The ACIP estimated that approximately 24 million persons would be included in phase 1a. This included approximately 21 million HCP who worked in settings such as hospitals, outpatient clinics, and community offices, emergency medicine providers, home healthcare, pharmacies, public health clinics, staffed LTCFs, and more.

Given supply constraints, initially, many states sub-prioritized phase 1a to focus on HCP most involved in care of COVID-19 patients and those who provide care for critically ill individuals.

As supplies have increased, most states have been able to broaden distribution to more groups within phase 1a.

Phase 1b consists of approximately 49 million persons and includes frontline essential workers who did not work in health-care, as well as persons >= 75 years of age. Essential workers are those who perform tasks critical for society functioning and include first responders (e.g., police and firefighters), food and agriculture workers, US postal service workers, workers in man-ufacturing facilities, grocery store workers, persons who work in public transit, school and education persons including teachers and school staff, and childcare workers.

Phase 1c consists of an estimated additional 129 million per-sons and includes all persons 65–74 years, persons 16–64 years with medical conditions that increase the risk of severe COVID-19, and other workers considered essential, including workers in transportation, water and wastewater, food service, shelter and housing, finance, information technology and communications, energy, legal, media, public safety, and public health workers. The list of high-risk medical conditions is long and consists of adults of any age with the following conditions: cancer; chronic kidney dis-ease; chronic obstructive pulmonary disease (COPD); heart condi-tions, such as heart failure, coronary artery disease, or cardiomy-opathies; immunocompromised state (weakened immune system) from solid organ transplant; obesity (body mass index [BMI] $\geq$30 kg/m^2 but <40 kg/m^2); severe obesity (BMI $\geq$40 kg/m^2); sickle cell disease; smoking; type 2 diabetes mellitus; and pregnancy.[1]

---

1 "The Advisory Committee on Immunization Practices' Updated Interim Recommendation for Allocation of COVID-19 Vaccine - United States, December 2020." Centers for Disease Control and Prevention, December 31, 2020. https://www.cdc.gov/mmwr/volumes/69/wr/mm695152e2.htm?s _cid=mm695152e2_w.

Phase 2 consists of all remaining adults and adolescents >=16 years of age. At the time of this writing, no COVID-19 vaccines were approved for use in children. Studies are underway to assess safety and effectiveness in children.

Recommendations for use

The ACIP has recommended the Pfizer-BioNTech COVID 19 for all persons >=16 years of age without contraindications to vaccination.[2] Two doses of 0.3 ml are recommended three weeks (21 days) apart. A second dose administered 17 days or longer after the first dose is acceptable. A second dose administered more than three weeks after dose 1 is acceptable, and delay in receipt does not necessitate restarting the vaccine schedule. No further doses are recommended at this time.

The ACIP recommended the Moderna vaccine for all persons >=18 years without contraindications. Two doses of 0.5 ml are recommended separated by an interval of four weeks (28 days). Intervals between doses as short as 24 days apart are acceptable. Like the Pfizer-BioNTech vaccine, intervals longer than the recommended interval are acceptable. There is no need to restart the series if the interval is longer.

While both vaccines are made with mRNA and have a lipid coat, it is recommended that both doses be the same product. Thus, if the first dose is Pfizer-BioNTech, the second dose should be the same brand. The Moderna vaccine should not be used. However, if a person receives one dose of one of the vaccines and a second

---

2 "Interim Clinical Considerations for Use of MRNA COVID-19 Vaccines." Centers for Disease Control and Prevention, January 21, 2021. https://www .cdc.gov/vaccines/covid-19/info-by-product/clinical-considerations.html.

dose of another vaccine, no further doses are recommended at this time.

The ACIP recommends that the mRNA COVID-19 vaccines be administered without any other vaccines at an interval of 14 days before or after other vaccines to be given or have been given. If it turns out that other vaccines were administered within this interval, there is no need to repeat doses of the COVID-19 vaccines or the other vaccines. In situations in which there is urgent need for other vaccines within a few days of COVID-19 vaccines (e.g., need for tetanus toxoid for a wound), those vaccines should be administered.

At the present time, there are no recommendations for further booster doses of the Moderna or Pfizer vaccines. The duration of immunity is not known but is being evaluated. Should there be a decrease in immunity over time, boosters would likely be recommended at an interval based on when there is a significant decrease in immunity.

Persons who have had a SARS-CoV-2 infection should be vaccinated. This is because there are persons who have had such infections who later developed a second infection. While there is no specified interval between the SARS-CoV-2 infection and when COVID-19 vaccines can be administered, it may be reasonable to delay vaccination until the vaccinee is fully recovered from the COVID-19 illness. Second infections with SARS-CoV-2 are very uncommon in the 90 days after the initial infection.

COVID-19 vaccines are generally not recommended to prevent infection with SARS-CoV-2 in persons who were already exposed to the virus. That's because the incubation period from exposure to onset of disease is most commonly 4–5 days, not enough time for a protective immune response to be developed following vaccination.

COVID-19 vaccines should be administered to persons with underlying medical conditions that increase their risk of more severe COVID-19. Further, vaccination can be performed in persons whose immune systems are compromised, provided they have no contraindications. However, such persons should be informed that it is currently unclear if they will make a protective immune response. Thus, they should continue to implement non-pharmaceutical interventions (masking, social distancing, and frequent hand washing).

Persons with autoimmune disorders, such as rheumatoid arthritis, can be vaccinated. However, there are no data currently evaluating the safety and efficacy in such individuals.

Pregnant women appear to have an increased risk of severe COVID-19. Information is available from animal studies for the mRNA and other vaccine platforms and the data do not show adverse effects on the pregnant animal or the offspring. Because the mRNA vaccines are not "live," experts believe these vaccines will **not** have deleterious effects on the pregnant woman or her offspring. However, there are limited data demonstrating the safety and efficacy of the mRNA vaccines in pregnant women and only a small number of pregnant women have received mRNA vaccines. One advantage of mRNA vaccines is that while the mRNA enters cells, it is degraded rapidly and does not reach the nucleus of the cell where the DNA is located. Pregnant women considering vaccination should discuss the risks and benefits with their providers. Certainly, women planning to become pregnant who are recommended to receive the vaccine should be encouraged to complete their vaccination series prior to conception to ensure that they are maximally protected prior to pregnancy. American College of Obstetricians and Gynecologists (ACOG) recommends that women who are recommended to receive a COVID-19 vaccine should be offered the vaccine regardless of pregnancy status. The mRNA vaccines are not contraindicated in pregnancy, and pregnancy testing should not be a requirement for COVID-19 vaccination. Lactating persons should also be offered vaccine.

CONTRAINDICATIONS

The CDC lists three major contraindications to receipt of the mRNA COVID-19 vaccine.[3]

1. Severe allergic reaction (e.g., anaphylaxis) after a previous dose of an mRNA COVID-19 vaccine or any of its components
2. Immediate allergic reaction of any severity to a previous dose of an mRNA COVID-19 vaccine or any of its components (including polyethylene glycol [PEG])*
3. Immediate allergic reaction of any severity to polysorbate (due to potential cross-reactive hypersensitivity with the vaccine ingredient PEG)*

---

3 "Interim Clinical Considerations for Use of MRNA COVID-19 Vaccines." Centers for Disease Control and Prevention, January 21, 2021. https://www .cdc.gov/vaccines/covid-19/info-by-product/clinical-considerations.html #Contradictions.

*These persons should not receive mRNA COVID-19 vaccination (Pfizer-BioNTech or Moderna) at this time unless they have been evaluated by an allergist-immunologist and it is determined that the person can safely receive the vaccine (e.g., under observation, in a setting with advanced medical care available).

Anaphylaxis (an-a-fi-LAK-sis) (see also Chapter 5) is a serious allergic response that often involves swelling, hives, lowered blood pressure, and, in severe cases, shock. If anaphylactic shock isn't treated immediately, it can be fatal.[4]

A major difference between anaphylaxis and other allergic reactions is that anaphylaxis typically involves more than one system of the body. Symptoms usually start within five to 30 minutes of coming into contact with an allergen to which an individual is allergic. Warning signs may include:

- Red rash (usually itchy and may have welts/hives)
- Swollen throat or swollen areas of the body
- Wheezing
- Passing out
- Chest tightness
- Trouble breathing
- Hoarse voice
- Trouble swallowing
- Vomiting
- Diarrhea
- Stomach cramping
- Pale or red color to the face and body

---

4 "Anaphylaxis: AAAAI." The American Academy of Allergy, Asthma & Immunology. Accessed February 2, 2021. https://www.aaaai.org/conditions-and-treatments/conditions-dictionary/anaphylaxis.

As noted, the incidence of anaphylaxis with COVID-19 vaccines is quite low. In surveillance since the introduction of these vaccines in December 2020 and widespread use, 2.5 cases of anaphylaxis per million doses occurred with the first dose of the Moderna COVID-19 vaccine administered and five cases per million doses administered after receipt of the first dose of the Pfizer-BioNTech vaccine. A strong female predominance of anaphylaxis case reports exists for both vaccines. Some individuals with anaphylaxis had a history of allergies or allergic reactions, including to drugs, contrast media, and foods or had experienced an episode of anaphylaxis in the past not associated with receipt of a vaccine. No clear geographic clustering of anaphylaxis cases has been observed, and the cases occurred after receipt of doses from multiple vaccine lots. Locations that administer vaccines should have the necessary supplies and trained staff available to manage anaphylaxis, implement postvaccination observation periods, immediately treat persons experiencing anaphylaxis signs and symptoms with intramuscular injection of epinephrine, and transport patients to facilities where they can receive advanced medical care.

PRECAUTIONS TO VACCINATION WITH MRNA COVID-19 VACCINES

Persons who have experienced an immediate allergic reaction to any non-COVID-19 vaccine or an injectable therapy (e.g., antibiotics given by injection in the arm) are considered to have a precaution to vaccination with mRNA COVID-19 vaccines. Whether such persons are at risk of developing a severe reaction to COVID-19 vaccines is unknown. Such persons should discuss whether they should receive a COVID-19 vaccine with their healthcare provider. Factors to be considered in weighing the risks and benefits of COVID-19 vaccination include the risk of exposure to SARS-CoV-2, risk of severe disease if infected, whether the person has been previously infected with SARS-CoV-2, and the ability to be vaccinated, if the benefits are judged to outweigh the risks, in a setting in which appropriate medical care is immediately available. These individuals should wait 30 minutes after vaccination at the vaccine site to monitor for the onset of symptoms of anaphylaxis.

DISTRIBUTION PLAN FOR VACCINES

In the United States, the federal government has entered into agreements with the vaccine manufacturers to buy vaccines to cover most of the population. Since the vaccines will be purchased with taxpayer funds, the vaccine costs will be free for recipients. Providers of the vaccines can charge an administration fee. However, no one can be denied vaccine for inability to pay.[5] Vaccination providers can be reimbursed for this by the patient's public or private insurance company or, for uninsured patients, by the Health Resources and Services Administration's Provider Relief Fund.

The federal government is allocating vaccines to states based on the population of that state. By early February 2021, over 60 million doses of the the two EUA vaccines had been distributed to the states. The states then make decisions about distributing the

---

5 "Frequently Asked Questions about COVID-19 Vaccination." Centers for Disease Control and Prevention, January 25, 2021. https://www.cdc.gov/coronavirus/2019-ncov/vaccines/faq.html.

vaccine to providers within the state.[6] The vaccine distribution process[7] starts with filling and finishing by the manufacturers. States decide how vaccines will be distributed within their states. The Association of State and Territorial Health Officials (ASTHO) has developed a website that describes each state's distribution program.[8] These plans cover how the vaccine will be shipped, how it should be stored, and how it should be used to optimize safety and efficacy. In addition, the information provides guidance on how to enroll providers who will administer the vaccines.

The Pfizer-BioNTech mRNA vaccine requires storage in ultra-cold freezers between −80°C and −60°C (−112°F and −76°F) up to the expiration date.[9] There are thermal shipping containers using the Controlant Temperature Monitoring Device (TMD). The appropriate temperature is maintained by adding dry ice to the shipping container according to the manufacturer's guidance. When vaccines are received, they can be kept in refrigerators between 2°C and 8°C (36°F and 46°F) for up to five days (120 hours).

6 "Covid-19 Vaccines: FAQs." American Medical Association, accessed February 2, 2021. https://www.ama-assn.org/system/files/2020-12/covid-19 -vaccine-physician-faqs.pdf.

7 "Covid-19 Vaccines." U.S. Department of Health & Human Services, accessed February 2, 2021. https://www.hhs.gov/sites/default/files/ows-vaccine -distribution-process.pdf.

8 "ASTHO COVID-19 Jurisdictional Vaccination Plans Compendium." Association of State and Territorial Health Officials, December 10, 2020. https://www.astho.org/COVID-19/Jurisdictional-Vaccination-Plans -Compendium.

9 "Pfizer-BioNTech COVID-19 Vaccine Questions." Centers for Disease Control and Prevention, accessed February 2, 2021. https://www.cdc.gov/ vaccines/covid-19/info-by-product/pfizer/pfizer-bioNTech-faqs.html.

The Moderna mRNA vaccine does not require the same cold storage as the Pfizer-BioNTech mRNA vaccine.[10] Vaccines may be stored in a freezer between -25°C and -15°C (-13°F and 5°F). Vaccine vials may be stored in the refrigerator between 2°C and 8°C (36°F and 46°F) for up to 30 days before vials are punctured.

COVID-19 VACCINE HESITANCY

Multiple surveys have found a substantial proportion of the population is hesitant with regard to being willing to be vaccinated against COVID-19 with the available vaccines. This hesitancy in part relates to concerns the vaccines have not been adequately assessed for safety and efficacy as part of Operation Warp Speed (OWS), now the United States government effort. Further, there are concerns that the vaccines may be harmful. Among the hesitant, there is a range of beliefs from people who absolutely will never take the vaccines to people who want to wait and see what happens based on the initial people vaccinated.

Willingness to accept a SARS-CoV-2 vaccine varies by country. In an online survey of 13,426 participants from 19 countries who were asked if they would accept a "proven, safe and effective vaccine," 72% overall said they completely or somewhat agreed. The highest proportion of positive responses were from China, South Korea, and Singapore (over 80%), whereas the lowest were from Russia (55%).

---

10 "Moderna Covid-19 Vaccine Storage and Handling Summary." Centers for Disease Control and Prevention, accessed February 2, 2021. https://www .cdc.gov/vaccines/covid-19/info-by-product/moderna/downloads/storage -summary.pdf.

In the United States, in a survey of 991 individuals conducted in April 2020, 58% reported that they would accept a SARS-CoV-2 vaccine, 32% were unsure, and 11% would decline vaccination. Vaccine hesitancy was more likely among those who were younger (<60 years old), were Black, had not obtained a college degree, and/or had not received influenza vaccine in the prior year. Among those who said they would decline the vaccine, the most common reasons were the belief that they are not at risk for COVID-19 (57%), and lack of trust (33%). Among those who were unsure, the common reasons were specific concerns about the SARS-CoV-2 vaccine itself (57%) and the need for more information (25%). It has been proposed that vaccine acceptance might increase if vaccines were confirmed to be highly effective; in another United States survey, an increase in efficacy of the proposed vaccine from 50 to 90% was associated with a 10% higher mean willingness to receive it. However, in a poll in December 2020 as vaccine efficacy data of 95% were being presented, 47% of Americans were still hesitant to get a COVID-19 vaccine. The willingness to be vaccinated was tightly linked to whether the individuals trusted the safety and efficacy of the vaccines.

More recently, the Institute for Health Metrics and Evaluation (IHME) of the University of Washington displayed willingness to accept COVID-19 vaccines by state using data as of January 8, 2021 (Figure 8, page 119). As noted in most states, only about 50% of persons would be willing to accept a COVID-19 vaccine, and more than 20% would reject such vaccines. The remainder would take a "wait and see" attitude before accepting or completely rejecting vaccines.

As detailed earlier in Chapters 4 and 5, corners have not been cut in the studies required to assess vaccine safety and efficacy of COVID-19 vaccines. The phase 3 trials conducted have included 30,000 or more participants with approximately half receiving vaccines and the other half receiving placebo. What has been sped up is the time frame going from phase 1 clinical trials to the trials used to get FDA approval, the phase 3 trials, as well as the federal government committing to manufacturers of the vaccines to purchase vaccines in parallel with clinical trials testing. The CDC has prepared excellent materials to help healthcare providers explain to the public what has been done to assure available COVID-19 vaccines are both safe and effective.[11]

Building confidence among persons eligible for COVID-19 vaccination is important not only to protect themselves but also to protect community, which includes persons not recommended for vaccination (e.g., children, persons with medical contraindications). These persons are indirectly protected if there is high immunity to COVID-19 in the community (i.e., herd immunity) that prevents them from being exposed to the virus. High immunity to COVID-19 breaks the chain of human-to-human transmission.

---

11 "Building Confidence in Covid-19 Vaccines Among Your Patients." Centers for Disease Control and Prevention, accessed February 2, 2021. https://www.cdc.gov/vaccines/covid-19/downloads/VaccinateWConfidence-TipsForHCTeams_508.pdf.

Figure 8: Percentage of all adults who would reject, accept, or are unsure about receiving the vaccine by state and DC, US

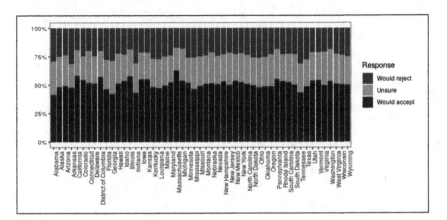

Figure 6: Percentage of all adults who would reject or opt to be immunized against receiving the vaccine by state and DC, US

Chapter 8

Summary

As the SARS-Cov2 virus emerged and spread globally in early 2020, unprecedented national and international efforts began to develop and test vaccines to control the devastating pandemic. This book reviews the remarkable progress in developing COVID-19 vaccines, the amazing effectiveness of the early vaccines, and the huge challenges of delivering them to the population. To put this extraordinary progress into perspective, the history of other vaccines is presented and the roles of vaccines in establishing individual protection and protection of the community, "vaccines that protect the unvaccinated" is explained. The rigorous processes whereby vaccines are evaluated in distinct phases and the steps that must be met prior to obtaining regulatory approval for both vaccine safety and effectiveness are highlighted. The multiple vaccine approaches to COVID-19 vaccines are reviewed, and new vaccine approaches such as "messenger" or mRNA vaccine that may revolutionize future vaccine development are discussed. The comprehensive models used to provide recommendations and priorities for vaccination of groups of people at risk are also summarized. We also review the need of careful assessments to address questions after the vaccines are approved. These include duration of immunity, risk factors for vaccine failure, impact of viral evolution and variant strains, and assessment of both immediate and long-term safety. Overcoming concerns about vaccine acceptance is a key issue. The work is not finished, second-generation vaccines are in human trials, safety and immunogenicity in children and pregnancy need to be established, variant viruses are emerging, and the duration of protection of these vaccines remains to be defined.

United States Emergency Use Authorization (EUA) Approved Vaccines

---

MRNA VACCINES (FDA VRBPAC BRIEFINGS, DEC 2021):

PFIZER-BIONTECH:

The Pfizer-BioNTech COVID-19 vaccine is a white to off-white sterile, preservative-free, frozen suspension for intramuscular injection. The vaccine contains a nucleoside-modified messenger RNA (modRNA) encoding the viral spike glycoprotein (S) of SARS-CoV-2. The vaccine also includes the following ingredients: lipids, potassium chloride, monobasic potassium phosphate, sodium chloride, dibasic sodium phosphate dihydrate, and sucrose (Table 3). The Pfizer-BioNTech COVID-19 Vaccine is supplied as a frozen [between −80°C to −60°C (−112°F to −76°F)] multi-dose (five-dose) vial. The vaccine must be thawed and diluted in its original vial with 1.8 mL of sterile 0.9% sodium chloride injection, USP prior to administration. After dilution, the vial contains five or six doses of 0.3 mL per dose. After dilution, the multiple-dose vials must be stored between 2°C–25°C (35°F–77°F) and used within six hours from the time of dilution. The Pfizer-BioNTech COVID-19 Vaccine, BNT162b2 (30 μg) is administered intramuscularly (IM) as a series of two 30 μg doses (0.3 mL each) 21 days apart.

MODERNA:

The Moderna COVID-19 vaccine is a white sterile, preservative-free, frozen suspension for injection into the upper arm muscle. The vaccine contains a synthetic messenger ribonucleic acid (mRNA) encoding the stabilized (called the pre-fusion) spike protein (S) of the SARS-CoV-2 virus that causes COVID-19. The vaccine also contains the following ingredients: lipids (at a ratio of 50:10:38.5:1.5), salts, buffers and sugar (Table 3, page 125). The Moderna COVID-19 vaccine is provided as a frozen suspension in multi-dose vial containing 10 doses of 100 ug /per dose. The vaccine is thawed prior to administration. After thawing, a maximum of 10 doses can be withdrawn from each vial. Vials can be stored refrigerated for up to 30 days prior to first use. The Moderna COVID-19 Vaccine, mRNA-1273 (100 μg) is administered intramuscularly as a series of two doses (0.5 mL each), given 28 days apart.

The complete FDA briefing documents that contributed to Emergency Use Authorization for these mRNA vaccines are found at www.fda.gov/media/144245/download and www.fda.gov/media/144434/download.

Table 3.

Ingredients* included in mRNA COVID-19 vaccines

Description	Pfizer-BioNTech	Moderna
mRNA	Nucleoside-modified mRNA encoding the viral spike (S) glycoprotein of SARS-CoV-2	Nucleoside-modified mRNA encoding the viral spike (S) glycoprotein of SARS-CoV-2
Lipids	2[(polyethylene glycol)-2000]-N,N-ditetradecylacetamide	PEG2000-DMG: 1,2-dimyristoyl-rac-glycerol, methoxypolyethylene glycol
	1,2-distearoyl-sn-glycero-3-phosphocholine	1,2-distearoyl-sn-glycero-3-phosphocholine
	Cholesterol	Cholesterol
	(4-hydroxybutyl)azanediyl) bis(hexane-6,1-diyl) bis(2-hexyldecanoate)	SM-102: heptadecan-9-yl 8-((2-hydroxyethyl) (6-oxo-6-(undecyloxy) hexyl) amino) octanoate
Salts, sugars, buffers	Potassium chloride	Tromethamine
	Monobasic potassium phosphate	Tromethamine hydrochloride
	Sodium chloride	Acetic acid
	Dibasic sodium phosphate dihydrate	Sodium acetate
	Sucrose	Sucrose

* Neither vaccine contain eggs, gelatin, latex, or preservatives.

Note: Both the Pfizer-BioNTech and Moderna COVID-19 vaccines contain polyethylene glycol (PEG). PEG is a primary ingredient in osmotic laxatives and oral bowel preparations for colonoscopy procedures, an inactive ingredient or excipient in many medications, and is used in a process called pegylation to improve the therapeutic activity of some medications (including certain chemotherapeutics). Additionally, cross-reactive hypersensitivity between PEG and polysorbates (included as an excipient in some vaccines and other therapeutic agents) can occur.[1]

---

1   "Interim Clinical Considerations for Use of MRNA COVID-19 Vaccines." Centers for Disease Control and Prevention, January 21, 2021. https://www .cdc.gov/vaccines/covid-19/info-by-product/clinical-considerations.html

Acknowledgments: We want to again recognize the global scientific contributions to the development of COVID-19 vaccines. We thank the contributions of Julie McElrath MD PhD for contributions to COVID-19 immunology (Stephens DS and McElrath, MJ, COVID-19 Path to Immunity; *JAMA*, 2020;324(13):1279–1281, 2021): Michael Konomos, MS CMI, Lead Medical Illustrator and Satyen Tripathi, Visual Medical Education, Emory School of Medicine; and Dianne Watson for administrative support. A special thanks to Dianne Miller for administrative support and coordination in assembling this book.

Conflicts of Interest: Drs. Orenstein, Edwards and Stephens are supported by research awards including UM1AI148684 (Emory University) from the National Institute of Allergy and Infectious Disease (NIAID) and are members of the NIAID Infectious Diseases Clinical Research Consortium–Vaccine and Treatment Evaluation Units. Dr. Stephens is a coleader of the COVID Prevention Network (CoVPN). Dr. Orenstein is on the Scientific Advisory Board for Moderna. Dr. Edwards is a consultant to IBM and Bionet and on the Data Safety and Monitoring Boards of Pfizer, Sanofi, Merck, Roche, X-4 Pharma, Seqirus, and Moderna.

Disclaimer: The conclusions in this report are those of the authors and do not necessarily represent views of the respective institutions or the National Institutes of Health or other federal agencies.

Index